Where Two Worlds Touch

A Spiritual Journey Through Alzheimer's Disease

Jade C. Angelica

Skinner House Books
Boston

Copyright © 2014 by Jade C. Angelica. All rights reserved. Published by Skinner House Books, an imprint of the Unitarian Universalist Association of Congregations, a liberal religious organization with more than 1,000 congregations in the U.S. and Canada, 25 Beacon St., Boston, MA 02108-2800.

www.skinnerhouse.org

Printed in the United States

Cover and text design by Suzanne Morgan
Front cover and frontispiece photos by Coleen Hein

print ISBN: 978-1-55896-711-3 / eBook ISBN: 978-1-55896-712-0

6 5 4 3 2 1 / 15 14 13

Library of Congress Cataloging-in-Publication Data
Angelica, Jade C. (Jade Christine), 1952-
Where two worlds touch : a spiritual journey through Alzheimer's disease / Jade Angelica.
   pages cm
Includes bibliographical references.
   ISBN 978-1-55896-711-3 (pbk. : alk. paper)—ISBN 978-1-55896-712-0 (ebook) 1. Alzheimer's disease—Patients—Care. 2. Alzheimer's disease—Patients—Biography. 3. Aging parents—Care—Religious aspects. I. Title.
   RC523.A54 2014
   616.8'31—dc23
          2013021505

We are grateful for permission to reprint the following copyrighted material:

"Facts and Figures about Alzheimer's and Dementia," adapted from Alzheimer's Association website, alz.org. Used with permission of the Alzheimer's Association.

Adaptation of "Yes, Virginia, There Is a Santa Claus," by Jade Angelica, in *The Journal of Pastoral Care and Counseling*, Vol. 65, No. 2 (2011), 10:1-2. Used with permission of *The Journal of Pastoral Care and Counseling*.

Adaptation of "Elephant and the Blind Men" from *Jain World*, www.jainworld.com/education/stories25.asp. Used with permission of Jain World.

"The Wind of the Spirit" by Myra Scoval. Used with permission of the poet's heirs.

"How Shall I?" by Libbie Deverich Stoddard. Used with permission of the author.

Excerpts from "Don't Go Back to Sleep," "The Guest House," and "The Most Alive Moment" by Rumi, translated by Coleman Barks. Used with permission of the translator.

Excerpt from the Penguin publication *The Subject Tonight Is Love: Sixty Wild and Sweet Poems of Hafiz*, copyright 1996 and 2002 by Daniel Ladinsky and used with his permission.

Letter to the Alzheimer's Association by Sol Rogers. Used with permission of the author.

"Theses on Healing (and Cure)" by Fred Reklau, from *Partners in Care: Medicine and Ministry Together*, used by permission of the author and Wipf and Stock Publishers, www.wipfandstock.com

"Gott spricht zu jedem.../God speaks to each of us...," from RILKE'S BOOK OF HOURS: LOVE POEMS TO GOD by Rainer Maria Rilke, translated by Anita Barrows and Joanna Macy, translation copyright © 1996 by Anita Barrows and Joanna Macy. Used by permission of Riverhead Books, an imprint of Penguin Group (USA) LLC.

All the stories in this book about Alzheimer's are true and are based either on my observations and recollections or on caregiver interviews and conversations. In some cases, names and certain details have been changed according to family members' requests for privacy.

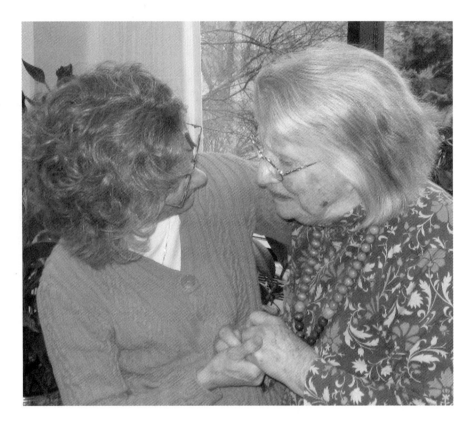

In honor and memory of my mom, Jeanne Marie, this work is dedicated to the beautiful, enlivened souls who have Alzheimer's disease and to all those who love and care for them. You are my inspiration.

—JA

About the
Healing Moments Alzheimer's Ministry

The primary mission of Healing Moments is to improve the quality of life for persons with Alzheimer's and their loved ones by enlivening their hearts with hope and enhancing their belief that meaningful relationships remain possible. Additional goals include: increasing caregiver knowledge, reducing caregiver stress, improving caregiver satisfaction, and decreasing conflict.

Founded in 2007 and offering programs throughout North America in a variety of settings—health care and nursing home facilities, retirement centers, conferences, retreat centers, religious congregations, colleges and universities, nursing schools, and seminaries—Healing Moments programs help professional and family caregivers understand and accept the diseases of dementia, and provide methods and motivation for developing effective skills for communicating, connecting, and caregiving. Using state-of-the-art teaching techniques, including spiritual practices and improvisational theater exercises, the programs are experiential, interactive, informative, inspiring, life-changing, and fun!

Programs include compassionate workshops for family and informal caregivers, dementia care training for professional caregivers, conference presentations, services of healing and remembrance for congregations and communities, and workshops for pastors, parish nurses, and pastoral care teams.

In 2010, Healing Moments received a First Place Best Practices for Older Adults Award from the National Council on Aging/National Interfaith Coalition on Aging.

For more information, visit www.healingmoments.org

To schedule a program, contact
Rev. Dr. Jade Angelica at jadeangelica@gmail.com or
Rev. Laura Randall at revlaurarandall@gmail.com

Contents

Looking Back, Walking On

Resources for Caregivers

Foreword

A shift of perception can transform our lives in ways we would not have imagined possible. When we see things differently we can act differently and we are freed to receive love and be more compassionate and loving.

I remember one Sunday, long ago, I was on my way to church on the subway in Philadelphia, reading and editing my sermon that I was to give that morning. I was wrapped up in my world, my worry, my self-preoccupation about how it would go. Yet I was forced to look up from my manuscript when a man walked onto the train at the next stop. He was very dirty, with at least a three-day-old beard. He generally had the appearance and smell of someone you hoped would sit elsewhere. As he entered the train, he said, "Good morning, Sally and John. Good morning." People gave him a quick glance, but no one spoke to him. At the next stop, as people got on, he called out again and again in a most cheerful voice, "Hi Robert and Janette, Peter and Diane."

Still, no one looked. At the next stop he did the same thing. Once again, silence.

At the next stop, same thing. Again silence. Then, all of a sudden, he plopped himself down in front of me and said, "I recognize everyone, no one recognizes me."

Finally I got it, and put down my sermon to turn to this man. I began by asking him his name.

"Bernie." he said, "What's yours?"

"Brita."

"Brita," he said, "do you know what?"

"No, Bernie. What?"

"You and I are twins. Yes, you and I are twins."

A bit taken aback, I replied, "Twins."

I did not exactly see a great similarity between us and obviously had been more attuned to our differences than our similarities. Then he looked at me and said, with a great big smile, "Yes, twins. You see, we both have two eyes, two ears, and a mouth. That makes us twins."

A moment later, the subway stopped and Bernie got up and walked out the door. It was an epiphany, an awakening that began that moment and has been working on me ever since. My encounter with Bernie began to teach me the most important lesson of my life: Only those who see their unity with all, truly see. Separation is an illusion that takes most of our lives from which to awake.

Few works I have read in my life have had such a profound impact on me as *Where Two Worlds Touch: A Spiritual Journey through Alzheimer's Disease*. My perception of Alzheimer's took a shift of seismic proportions after I read it, deepening the epiphany that first occurred thirty-five years ago on a subway. This book has changed forever how I view persons with Alzheimer's. Like many in our society, prior to reading *Where Two Worlds Touch* I thought of Alzheimer's as the dark hole of non-relation, a world characterized by lack of connection and extreme isolation. If we cannot think, who are we? If we cannot remember, who are we? If we don't recognize others, how do we convey the significance of their presence? If we can't communicate rationally with words, how do we find a way to meet in a meaningful way? How can I relate to people with Alzheimer's, and how could others relate to me if I were to get Alzheimer's? How could I be faithful and loving to someone I loved who no longer recognized me?

The potential for Alzheimer's to strike me or someone I love has been a deep fear of mine, a fate I considered to be worse than death. The lens through which I viewed Alzheimer's was colored only with darkness and the most profound sense of loss.

Reading this book opened a window into a new world of understanding that transformed my fear and deepened my sense of the mystery of life. Alzheimer's doesn't obliterate another's humanity or dignity, if we have eyes and ears tuned to meet them where they are, rather than where we are or where we want them to be. Caring for people with Alzheimer's has as much potential to transform us as it does those who have Alzheimer's—a transformation that can take us reluctantly but powerfully into the very heart of surrender and love. But it takes a new set of eyes and a new way of learning to be with someone to enter the landscape where a profound and life changing meeting can still take place and where we discover Alzheimer's patients still have the capacity to give and receive love.

In this exquisite piece of writing, Jade Angelica has woven a tapestry of story, poetry, and spiritual and theological reflection with scientific and medical research in a way that will forever influence how you think about Alzheimer's—and even more importantly, how you relate to those with Alzheimer's. It is, first and foremost, a reflection for those who care for people with Alzheimer's. It will open your eyes, your heart, and your life, and you will find something shifting in you, a way of seeing that deepens your understanding of life in all its agony, mystery, and beauty. It is not Pollyanna-ish, it cannot take away the real grief and suffering people experience in all the losses associated with Alzheimer's. Yet it does open a way to stay in connection amid those losses.

Jade Angelica takes us on a deeply personal journey of caring for her mother from the initial diagnosis of Alzheimer's until her mother's death, a period of nearly ten years. Through Angelica's spiritual journey, we encounter the fear, the avoidance, the denial, the utter helplessness that strike most who love someone who has Alzheimer's. But she takes us beyond the fear and avoidance, realizing that these are largely the result of not knowing how to be with someone who has Alzheimer's. She takes our hands and leads us through doors of new perception as we learn to live into a new mystery of being with a person who has Alzheimer's. Yes, it is true, a person with Alzheimer's, particularly someone in the more advanced stages, is not the person we knew. A wise friend once told me, "Love is the capacity to keep changing our perception of the other." To love someone with Alzheimer's requires a profound shift of perception, but not the shift so many often make—from a person to an empty shell, one with whom we can no longer share any meaningful relationship. Angelica opens our eyes to see how Alzheimer's patients have much to give and teach us about relationship; about being in the present moment; about communion, not just communication; about the practice of surrender and acceptance; about love; and about finding gratitude in unlikely places.

Through her background in improvisation, Angelica opens up a playful, fun, and brilliant means to be with Alzheimer's patients that allows us to learn the art of entering another's world. One who practices improvisation has to learn to respond creatively to the moment as it presents itself, accepting the offer extended by a partner, taking it as valid, and then saying or doing the next logical thing. This means accepting where the partner is right at that moment, saying yes to the moment, and joining them there, rather than contradicting them. Being with Alzheimer's patients requires going through the same process. We must learn the art of entering their world, figuring out their viewpoint, and taking it on for ourselves. It is intellectually and emotionally challenging work and can be immensely rewarding.

With 5.2 million Americans now diagnosed with Alzheimer's, and that number projected to reach 7.1 million by 2025, we must seek to cure what is now an incurable disease. Yet Alzheimer's reminds us that life will always be fragile, always marked by vulnerability and eventual diminishment. It reminds us that there are moments when any of us can become more or less helpless and must depend on the love and care of others.

Descartes had it all wrong when he said, "I think therefore I am." We are more than our rational faculties. Angelica is much closer to the truth when she writes, "I long to receive and give love, therefore I am." When we remember this—when we know in the marrow of our being that we were made for receiving and giving love from birth to death, no matter what— then we will know that we always belong to each other and that separation is an illusion. We only have to wake up to that fact again and again. Caring for those with Alzheimer's may be one of the best spiritual practices of our time for learning that only those who see their deep belonging, their unity with others, truly see. We have been blessed beyond measure with a wise and compassionate guide, Jade Angelica, to help us really meet persons with Alzheimer's, seeing them and ourselves with new eyes. And with this seeing, awakening to our deep belonging to one another.

Brita L. Gill-Austern
Austin Philip Guiles Professor of Psychology
    and Pastoral Theology
Andover Newton Theological School

Introduction

More than twenty years ago, early in my ministry education, I was given the rare opportunity to enroll in a doctoral course at Andover Newton Theological School. This course, Healing Is Meeting: The Vision of Martin Buber, taught by Professor Brita Gill-Austern, informed my worldview and planted seeds for transformation that have blossomed in various manifestations throughout my life. Years later, with Buber's insights still imprinted in my mind and heart, I encountered Alzheimer's disease. It was then that enrolling in this course appeared to be more like fate than mere opportunity.

Like most people, I was frightened to engage with Alzheimer's. My mother's diagnosis in 2001, however, beckoned me across the threshold into her mysterious world. There, seeds of transformation sprouted, and in many ways, Mom and I met each other for the first time.

Inspired by Buber, the message for caregivers in *Where Two Worlds Touch* is about the power and potential of true encounter. The message is related through the endearing and enlightening meetings I experienced with Mom, but this book is about more than our relationship. It's about meeting persons with Alzheimer's and falling into love and respect for them. It's about meeting caregivers who have learned to bear the unbearable, who demonstrate that it's okay—even desirable—to commit to caregiving even if it means *our* lives must change. It's about recognizing our limits as individuals and the failure of science to cure this disease. It's about accepting our frustrations and suffering, and then opening our hearts to hope and healing as we face a degenerative terminal disease. It's about the tender responsibility of becoming the legal guardian for a person who is completely helpless, and then struggling with awesome decisions about life and death. It's about grappling with the realities of Alzheimer's disease and the impact of these realities on families and science. It's about caregivers telling our stories and meeting scientists who will listen and help us change the world of Alzheimer's care. It's about seeing our selves and our humanity —our feelings, thoughts, reactions, and beliefs—through the lens of Alzheimer's. And it's about discovering life-giving possibilities in every corner of life.

Where Two Worlds Touch is like a tapestry, woven together by poetry and stories drawn from my experiences and those of other Alzheimer's caregivers, informed by literature in the Alzheimer's field of research, and grounded by spiritual and theological resources. The meetings between Mom and me anchor the universal aspects of my message within individual lives. The overall purpose of *Where Two Worlds Touch* is to remind us of the inherent dignity and worth of all persons—even persons with cognitive decline—and to remind us that interconnectedness is a central aspect of being human. We are not separate from persons with Alzheimer's. Our lives are woven together, and we are on this journey together.

Although this book is the culmination of many years of academic study, the information is presented in a style designed to open hearts and engage the spiritual imagination of readers as well as to be intellectually enlightening. The writing style is intended to be accessible for a general audience of family and professional Alzheimer's caregivers, with the goal of sharing forward the wisdom and comfort I have received from many teachers and companions. For those readers interested in the more academic aspects of my study of Alzheimer's care, including brain science and current research, detailed references are located in the Resources and Notes sections.

Although my intention is to comfort and accompany caregivers on the journey through Alzheimer's, my experience and interpretation may not speak to or comfort all caregivers, especially those who are grieving the loss of a loved one with Alzheimer's who is still living. My story is not one of losing my mother while she was living with Alzheimer's. Accordingly, my reflections do not focus on what was lost. They focus on what was found: my openness to discovering new possibilities, a deep relationship with my mother, and unconditional love flowing between us. Implementing improvisational theater techniques to effectively communicate and connect with, and care for persons with Alzheimer's is one of the unique discoveries I made and describe in this book.

One caregiving setting specifically addressed is the nursing home. For caregivers approaching the need to move their loved ones to assisted living or nursing home facilities, it's important to appreciate the difficulties surrounding this life change. It's an environment that caregivers may need to return to again and again until we can understand and accept that this is now our loved one's home. It's important to be gentle with ourselves during this transition but also to be committed and disciplined in our efforts to overcome any resistance.

For more than nine years, I have been immersed in rich learning about Alzheimer's care. Combining my personal encounter with Alzheimer's with my academic inquiry and my training and experience as a spiritual director, I write as a spiritual companion for family caregivers and anyone who loves someone with Alzheimer's. *Where Two Worlds Touch* reveals the experience of caregiving through the lens of a spiritual journey that has the potential to lead us through Alzheimer's into healing and wholeness. By embracing persons with Alzheimer's with open hearts, holy vision, and healing presence, it's possible that caregivers on this sacred journey will bear witness to the transforming power of Alzheimer's, as I did. It's also possible that caregivers will notice and receive unexpected gifts, and experience awe and gratitude for the ways that Alzheimer's can touch our hearts and transform our lives.

The topics and issues are presented and discussed in the context of spirituality, and the words *God* and *spirit* are used often. Understanding that these words have various meanings for people, I use them in a generic way not specific to any religious tradition. For me, these words represent an experiential reality of what is sacred, and they have deep meaning in my life. Theologian Marcus Borg's description resonates with my understanding of these words. He says that words used to describe the sacred represent a "strong sense of there being more to reality than the tangible world of our ordinary experience." Sacred words from various traditions (to include *God*, *Yahweh*, *Brahman*, *Atman*, *Allah*, the *Tao*, and *Great Spirit*) are "understood as that nonmaterial reality or presence that is experienced in extraordinary moments. . . . *The sacred (or numinous)* refers to the other reality that is encountered in these experiences."[1]

As part of my research, I interviewed family caregiver Mary Anne. Recently, Mary Anne and I met for lunch. The day before, she had read the story I wrote about her relationship with her mother, Ione, to her husband. He asked if what I wrote were my words or Mary Anne's. They were her words, of course. He expressed some surprise about Mary Anne's self-awareness and her depth of feeling about her mother's illness and decline. Mary Anne replied, "It was really helpful to talk to Jade about what I was feeling. No one had asked me these questions, so I hadn't actually thought about it before." Since pondering these questions was so helpful to Mary Anne, I have included them in the section Reflection Questions. If other caregivers feel inspired to explore their own hearts and minds, they may choose to use these questions as a guide.

Self-awareness and self-care are critical components in the lives of Alzheimer's caregivers, particularly family caregivers who are at heightened risk for health problems and depression due to stress. In addition to learning about Alzheimer's and developing specific external skills for self-care, such as relaxation and exercise, improving the internal skills of awareness and acceptance can lead to successful, satisfying caregiving experiences. The section Spiritual Practices includes introductory information about how caregivers can increase their awareness of themselves and others. Caregivers are strongly encouraged to give themselves permission to care for themselves as well as their loved ones.

My purpose for sharing my story and my discoveries is to reassure caregivers that they and their loved ones with Alzheimer's need not suffer in isolation or be overwhelmed by fear, loss, and responsibility on this journey. A cherished poem by Rainer Maria Rilke reflects the message of this book and reminds caregivers that we are not alone:

> God speaks to each of us as he makes us,
> then walks with us silently out of the night.
>
> These are the words we dimly hear:
>
> You, sent out beyond your recall,
> go to the limits of your longing.
> Embody me.
>
> Flare up like flame
> and make big shadows I can move in.

Let everything happen to you: beauty and terror.
Just keep going. No feeling is final.
Don't let yourself lose me.

Nearby is the country they call life.
You will know it by its seriousness.

Give me your hand.[2]

In the Beginning

The breeze at dawn has secrets to tell you,
Don't go back to sleep.
You must ask for what your really want,
Don't go back to sleep.
People are going back and forth across the doorsill
Where the two worlds touch.
The door is round and open,
Don't go back to sleep.

—Rumi

Three months after having hip replacement surgery, my mother Jeanne, then eighty-two, walked by herself to an appointment with her primary care doctor. That day she revealed a concern she was having about her memory. Indicating that memory loss was an early sign of Alzheimer's, the doctor prescribed a trial of Aricept.

Then Mom took what must have been a lonely walk home. About a mile in distance, this walk marked Mom's first steps on what became a ten-year journey through Alzheimer's disease.

Years later, as I read about this appointment in Mom's medical file, my heart was overcome by emotion. Aware of her lifelong aversion to doctors, I felt compassion for the humility it required for her to be open and vulnerable about her decline and to ask for help. I also felt admiration for her bravery in self-reporting this symptom, because she surely knew what it meant. Mom had cared for her older sister, who had died as a result of Alzheimer's ten years earlier. As I visualized her taking those first, solitary steps into Alzheimer's, the rightness of my decision to change my life and walk along with her during the final steps was reinforced yet again.

Every person's and every family's journey into Alzheimer's will begin, unfold, and end uniquely. Our histories, circumstances, fears, needs, and longings cohere into what our experience with Alzheimer's will become for us. Although there are infinite differences in the emotions and practicalities of caregiver experiences, the similarities of our sorrows and joys, the consistency of our struggles and victories, and those tiny unforgettable, forever cherished moments of connection with our loved ones are what will bind us together as we find our way along this mysterious path.

As we become your companions on this journey, Mom's spirit and I hope our story and our discoveries will bring comfort and inspiration to persons with Alzheimer's and caregivers. We hope our story will help families and communities develop a deeper understanding of dementia and nurture the belief that meaningful relationships remain possible throughout all the stages and diminishments of Alzheimer's.

Walking together, across the doorsill, into the world of Alzheimer's . . .

Awakening

Oblivion was my first companion on the Alzheimer's journey. I simply wasn't there to witness the beginning of Mom's decline.

We were separated geographically by twelve hundred miles. I lived in Maine, and Mom lived in Iowa. Complicated circumstances in both of our lives had prevented us from seeing each other for a few years. When we spoke on the phone, I didn't register any decline. I had always attributed oddities in Mom's memory, speech, or mood to drinking.

Twenty-five years earlier, I had begun separating emotionally from Mom. Before this, we had been very close, perhaps too close. As a child, I was her shadow, trying desperately to win her attention and approval. As a young adult, I had trouble identifying my own opinions, preferences, and needs, particularly if they seemed contrary to hers. In order to become my own person, I needed both geographic and emotional distance.

I also needed to protect myself from Mom's alcoholic lifestyle, judgmental nature, and limited worldview, which didn't allow me to choose sobriety or my own religious beliefs, to express vegetarian dietary preferences, or to speak my truth about what it was like for me growing up in an alcoholic, abusive home. Alcohol was the centerpiece of our family life and social gatherings, and my relationship with Mom became especially strained when I stopped drinking.

After Mom moved to the nursing home and I moved to Iowa to be her advocate, companion, and comforter, a relative criticized me for not spending more time with Mom during the years before Alzheimer's when she "could have appreciated" my presence. Although this criticism was hurtful to me, I realized that there was much this relative didn't understand about me, my family, my relationship with Mom, or my healing journey. Mom might have appreciated more visits from me during the years of separation, but possibly not. I was such a disappointment to her.

When I was in Iowa for my twenty-fifth high school reunion, the local paper wrote about my book on the moral emergency of child sexual abuse. Although neither book nor article revealed my personal history of abuse, Mom was shamed and threatened by what she perceived as public exposure. After reading the article in the morning paper, she flew into an alcohol-fueled rage. Her critical rants, echoing off the walls of her small house, culminated with the pronouncement, "I am not proud of you."

I was devastated.

By this time of my life, I had overcome my addictions to alcohol and drugs and had been sober for over fifteen years; I had graduated from Harvard Divinity School; I was an ordained minister (albeit not in Mom's religious tradition); I was doing a meaningful ministry on behalf of abused children and had published books and articles in the hopes of protecting them; I had received professional recognition and achieved a modest amount of financial security. By social standards, I had achieved some success. Although I had tried to please Mom by making deliberate and specific efforts to connect with her, in Mom's eyes and heart, I was a disappointment.

If modern theologian, Richard Rohr, is accurate in his belief about the spiritual journey that we have to leave home in order to actually find our way home,[1] it was precisely those years of geographic and emotional separation that allowed me to come home to Mom during her time of greatest need. My sibling had placed Mom in a nursing home and moved fifteen hundred miles away, so no one remained in Iowa to care for Mom. In my mind and heart, being abandoned and alone in a nursing home in the midst of diminishment from Alzheimer's disease was not an acceptable way for my mother to live the last years of her life.

I don't know if Mom ever did feel proud of me. However, her whole-souled smiles, her hugs and kisses, and her expressive sounds and admiring looks during the three and a half years we had together told me that she definitely appreciated my presence as her daily companion in the nursing home.

In 2002, when I learned from a cousin who saw Mom occasionally that signs of Alzheimer's were definitely present, avoidance became my next companion on the journey. Not denial, which is common for Alzheimer's family members, but avoidance. I knew Alzheimer's was among us. I knew because Alzheimer's had been a cloud over our family for nearly thirty years: Both of Mom's older sisters had some form of dementia, probably Alzheimer's. I still vividly remember the day in 1973 when dear Aunt Maggie wandered off during a family picnic in the small river town of Guttenberg, Iowa. She had gone to the restroom and never returned. In my photo collection there's a picture of her on that day, wearing my royal blue volleyball jacket and a bewildered smile.

That was the beginning for our family, and now, Maggie's daughter was telling me that Mom was showing signs of this disease. She encouraged me to read books about Alzheimer's, to watch videos and movies, and to explore the Alzheimer's Association website. I politely listened to her while consciously disguising my impatience, thanked her, and chose to avoid the entire subject. Fear, of course, was the foundation of my avoidance. David Shenk, a journalist who researched Alzheimer's disease and wrote *The Forgetting—Alzheimer's: Portrait of an Epidemic*, was also an avoider once. He helped me to feel forgiven for my avoidance and explained why this is a common reaction. "Opening the book, one fears, is tantamount to looking straight into the face of Alzheimer's—and perhaps one's own dark future. . . . So we avoid it. We don't read the books; we don't ask the questions; we don't visit our newly diagnosed neighbor. . . . It's only natural to not want to explore such awful thoughts."[2] Because Shenk and I have travelled through the valley of Alzheimer's avoidance, we wouldn't dare to judge others who are also following this path.

Avoidance was an effective companion for me—until 2003. Maggie's daughter made the thoughtful and gracious offer to bring Mom to Maine to visit me. Her offer was accompanied by the foreboding, "Before it's too late." And so I agreed. Mom was thrilled, as demonstrated by her packed suitcase ready and waiting by the door for two weeks before the trip. I was apprehensive.

To prepare myself for this visit from my mother and what I considered to be my first face-to-face meeting with Alzheimer's, I attended a personal growth workshop, one of many such experiences I had sought out during my twenty-plus years of healing. Influenced by the Episcopal priest Alan Jones to believe that the journey of our souls often presents itself in the form of a story,[3] I was especially intrigued when the workshop leader suggested that we could learn about our unconscious drives and longings by writing our life stories on one page.

I did this creative writing assignment eagerly and was impressed by my own poetic conciseness and my understanding of my life. Over dinner the night before Mom arrived, I told a friend about the workshop. Convinced that my one-page life story was well written and accurate, I read it to my friend with pride. It was a story of being vulnerable—as a child and as a woman—and being abused, abandoned, and betrayed by the very people who were entrusted with my care and safety. My friend looked at me in astonishment over the dinner table. Expecting praise, I was shocked by her reply. "You've done so much with your life, Jade. Why do you keep telling *that* story?"

The wisdom of my soul instantly knew the answer to her question: Because almost every part of my being, including my imagination, had been severely wounded by abusers in my childhood and my adult intimate relationships. Parts of me had healed, and other parts were continuing to heal. But my friend's question made me realize that I had closed down my imagination and shut myself off from seeing any new possibilities in my life story. Fortunately, this conversation opened my eyes and raised my awareness of this pattern just in time. A new possibility—in the form of my mother in decline from Alzheimer's disease—was about to step off a plane at the Portland airport and awaken my soul to an unimagined future.

Mom and her travelling companion, Maggie's daughter, arrived for a three-day visit in May. It's a breathtakingly beautiful time of year along Maine's southern coast, but Mom seemed to have eyes only for me. When she walked off the plane and caught sight of me, her face erupted into joy that radiated throughout her entire visit. She took my hand at the airport, and she didn't let go.

The changes in Mom were poignant, touching my heart in unexpected ways. One surprising change was that her judgmental nature seemed to be replaced by a kind of sweetness. It seemed that she had forgotten what a disappointment I had previously been to her. She called me her girl, smiled genuinely at me, and reached out to connect with me physically whenever possible.

Mom seemed curious about herself and her environment. There was a full-length mirror in the hallway of my apartment, and every time she passed the mirror, she paused at length to examine her reflection and comb her hair. Almost every picture from that trip shows Mom holding her comb in one hand. When I served our first lunch together, she was more interested in the silverware than in the food. She picked up her fork and looked closely at the handle. She turned it over, stroked it, and touched it to her cheek. In order to turn her attention away from the fork, I had to suggest that she taste her food. Not until much later did I realize the source of her fork fascination. When I first moved out on my own, Mom had given me this set of silver-plated flatware. It had belonged to *her* mother. This silverware, engraved with the initial *T*—the first letter of Mom's maiden name—was familiar from childhood. Unquestionably, some kind of recognition was happening for her.

Mom's surprising behaviors opened my heart and riveted my attention. I wanted to connect with her, to be supportive and caring, but it was clear that I didn't know what to do or how to be in her presence. I didn't know how to communicate with this transforming being, how to meet her needs, how to keep her safe, or how to navigate social practices such as dinner in a restaurant or attending a concert with someone who no longer understood—or practiced—conventional behaviors. One evening at a concert by a group of local a cappella singers, I had a flashback to a movie experience with my nephew when he was five. After fidgeting for a while, Mom started talking out loud. "Shhhh" didn't help. Finally Mom stood up, just as my nephew had, and shouted, just as my nephew had, "This is taking too long!" It was time to go.

My mom with Alzheimer's equaled a mystery to me, and the growing collection of things I didn't know, resulted in me feeling inadequate and afraid. My brief encounter with Mom during this phase of her disease opened my eyes and my heart to the helplessness that often overwhelms both persons with Alzheimer's and their caregivers. None of us knows what's happening, but whatever it is, we're not in control. And we don't know what to do about any of it.

During our time together in Maine, Mom and I were unconsciously planting the seeds for a new bond that would grow between us. Reading a letter that Mom wrote after returning to Iowa, it seemed as if my deepest desire, to be noticed and loved by her, was being fulfilled: "I'm more lonesome for you since visiting you," she wrote, "because you were especially nice to me. I never realized how caring you were." It was as if my mother were seeing me for the first time.

Over the next several months, we talked on the phone and wrote to each other regularly. I began to notice that my efforts to connect with Mom, which had previously been mostly obligatory and dreaded, were now expressed with enthusiasm and tenderness.

The damage to Mom's rational thinking somehow freed her to engage and communicate with me differently. Our phone interactions were uncomplicated yet deeply sincere. We talked about day-to-day activities. She was playing cribbage, walking the dog, feeding the birds, and planting flowers. I was learning to cook, walking alone by the ocean, and studying spiritual direction. A most significant change was that Mom listened to what I was saying; she really listened—without changing the subject in the middle of my sentences as she had throughout my life.

As we talked and wrote about plans to get together again, Mom even offered creative solutions for meeting my complicated health needs regarding travelling instead of criticizing me as she had in the past. This highlighted how much she wanted to be with me. Every precious interaction encouraged me, opened my heart further, and nourished our relationship.

Mom's letters, written on the teeniest stationery I'd ever seen (smaller than an index card), were simple and sweet. Using few words, she encouraged my endeavors and communicated honestly about her feelings. She was thrilled that I was studying spiritual direction. She probably didn't know what this was exactly, but she knew it was about getting closer to God. "I'm all for that!" she wrote repeatedly. She asked me to teach her how to concentrate when she prayed and how to deepen her relationship with God. She even expressed interest in my writing and asked me to send my articles to her. She had never done this. She apologized for making mistakes in her handwriting and sometimes wrote the same letter twice, copying it over to edit the mistakes and then sending both copies. Her awareness of her failing abilities and her efforts to send a nicely written letter touched me deeply. It seemed that Mom was building a home in my soul.

In her letters, she repeatedly thanked me for gifts I had sent, and I felt so grateful for her desire to appreciate me. She offered to send money to me for rent, probably recalling my financial troubles after my engagement had ended three years earlier. Although I didn't need the money at this time, her thoughtful effort to take care of me woke me up, and I began recognizing more and more of Mom's thoughtful efforts.

Having grown up on a farm, she loved plants and was a gifted gardener. She searched her seed books and found a special flower called Jade Eyes. She ordered the bulbs from a catalog, and when they arrived, she sent me the two biggest—presumably the heartiest, she said—to plant in my landlord's yard. She also planted two bulbs in her yard, so we would have "twins." The gorgeous blooms, puffs of tiny white flowers with very tiny jade green centers, came up in the spring in our yards in Maine and Iowa. Reaching across the miles that separated us, these blooms created a symbolic sense of connectedness.

Then Mom had a car accident and lost her driver's license. She was studying so hard, and taking and retaking the driver's test to get her license back. She wrote about this in every letter. The final failure—the doctor's statement that she was not competent to drive—was so painful for her. The compassion I felt for Mom's lost sense of freedom moved me to tears. It was the thorny threshold of her transformation from independence to dependence. She was beginning to understand that dependent people must often wait for their needs to be met, if they are met at all. She cried because she couldn't go to the grocery store when she wanted to. I cried too, wishing I were there to take her.

As Mom's letters arrived less frequently, our phone conversations awakened concerns within me for her welfare. For example, learning that she was taking Alzheimer's medication and still drinking heavily caused some worry. But I didn't realize exactly how dangerous this was because I had consistently and successfully avoided learning anything specific about Alzheimer's. A year later, when I accompanied Mom to doctors' appointments, I became enlightened about the potential perils of alcohol use by dementia patients.

A year after Mom's visit, I was startled awake in the night by a frightening dream about her failing health. I was sure something serious had happened to her. When I called her in the morning, my sibling told me a story that resurrected my panicked memories of that day in 1973 when Aunt Maggie had wandered away from the family picnic. My sibling had taken Mom camping in Minnesota. Mom had gone to use the restroom and departed from the campground with intention. She wasn't wandering aimlessly, as one might expect. State troopers found her walking on an interstate highway and she told them she was going "home to Dubuque." The next stop had been the hospital emergency room, where Mom was given antipsychotic drugs to calm her out-of-control emotions. The hospital report documents the anger and despair of a frightened, confused, and extremely vulnerable person.

Learning from this experience, my sibling realized that taking Mom on camping trips wasn't such a good idea. Since there was a similar trip planned later in the summer, I was asked to stay with Mom for those two weeks. Eager to spend time with her, I enthusiastically said, "Yes, of course I'll come!"

Then my sibling said that Mom had become uncooperative, describing her as angry and her behavior as volatile and combative. According to my sibling, Mom had no appetite and refused her medication as well as her meals. My sibling coached me to be stern if I wanted Mom to obey, suggesting that I raise my voice, threaten to take her to the mental hospital, or give her the antipsychotic medication prescribed by her doctor. Alarmingly, my sibling added that after Mom took the meds to calm down, she was kind of out of it for a few weeks. My enthusiasm drained away, and I was terrified. What had I said yes to?

In my heart, I knew there had to be a way to care for my vulnerable mother that didn't involve yelling, threatening, or giving medication that isn't even recommended for use by people with dementia. There *had* to be a better way, and my desire to find it catapulted me out of avoidance.

Intellectually and emotionally unprepared, and terrified by the mystery before me, I was nonetheless about to take my first steps on the journey through Alzheimer's.

Accepting and Improvising

To prepare myself for my upcoming trip into the unknown waiting for me in Iowa, I undertook a thorough search of the Alzheimer's Association website. I was specifically looking for information about how to interact with and care for Mom in ways that were gentler, more compassionate, and more effective. I didn't find anything particularly helpful, but I did encounter the terrifying details and statistics I had been carefully avoiding. The importance of my quest, however, motivated me to soldier on through my rising terror.

One night, as I talked on the phone to a colleague, my distress and confusion about Alzheimer's disease and being with Mom were highly evident. Offering compassionate, concrete caring for my heightened emotional state, my colleague recommended a new book, *Learning to Speak Alzheimer's*, by Joanne Koenig Coste.

When I hung up the phone, I immediately ordered it online and had it sent via overnight express. My first opportunity to begin reading it was on the plane en route to Iowa. I stepped onto American Airlines flight 409 in Portland, terrified about the mysterious world I was about to enter. As I stepped off that airplane three hours later in Chicago, I felt informed, inspired, and prepared to try out what seemed to be a much better way.

Joanne Koenig Coste had learned how to be an Alzheimer's caregiver by doing it. Shortly after the birth of her fourth child, she began caring for her husband, who was diagnosed with progressive dementia in his mid-forties. By sharing what she had discovered through her own experience, Coste, a renowned pioneer known for implementing positive methods of caring for persons with Alzheimer's, had become my first guide on this journey.

I was able to recognize Coste's wisdom only because, a few years earlier after my engagement ended, a friend observed that I could use some fun in my life. She suggested that I take a class in improvisational theater. Why I ever followed up on this idea is still baffling because I was not the improvisation type—not at all! I took the class though, and as my friend predicted, it was so much fun. Once I overcame my fear of not knowing what in the world was going on, I fell in love with the craft of improvisation, which I then studied and practiced for several years in Maine and in Boston.

Almost instantly, I noticed that improvisation, when practiced not as comedy but as an intentional method for increasing self-awareness, possessed tremendous potential for healing and transformation. Through this lens of improvisation, I read a section from *Learning to Speak Alzheimer's* that changed my life—and Mom's:

> The staff was busily opening draperies, letting the first beams of morning light into the rooms inhabited by the forty-five residents on floor two of the nursing center.
>
> "I want to see my mother," Mary said softly to no one in particular as she shuffled from her room, holding on to the wall.
>
> Claire, a young nurse's aide who happened to pass by at that moment, took Mary's hand. Then she said, sympathetically, "Mary, your mother has been dead a long time."

"Don't be so fresh," Mary said, pulling her hand away, "You don't know what you're talking about."

"Try to remember, Mary. You haven't seen your mother in years. She died when you were in your forties. You're eighty-seven now."

Mary shoved Claire out of her path. "My mother was right here this morning. We had breakfast together like always. Now get out of my way."

Gently, Claire took Mary's arm and began to guide her to the large-print calendar hanging in the nurses' station.

"No. I'm not going with you."

Claire tightened her grip. "I want to show you the date. Your mother died a long time ago."

Mary sputtered, "You—you—you—*hussy*." Then, swinging her free arm, Mary caught the aide with a backhand slap to the face. Claire called for help.

Her colleagues responded and quickly subdued Mary, injecting her with an antipsychotic medication. For the rest of the morning, the staff kept Mary restrained to a chair in front of the nurses' station, where they could see her.[4]

Reading this scenario, caused my breathing to freeze in a moment of fear, wondering if this was the kind of volatile behavior my sibling was experiencing with Mom. I started to breathe again as Coste analyzed the reasons for the conflict. The aide's response, she explained, was a form of "reality orientation," which attempts to bring a seemingly confused person back to the current time and place. Although still taught in nursing schools and widely recommended as an intervention for elders who are forgetful from time to time, Dr. Paul Raia does not recommend reality orientation for persons of any age with any kind of dementia. The cognitive decline that accompanies Alzheimer's increasingly limits the ability of persons with this disease to process information that contradicts their own mental understanding. Ignoring and/or dismissing their experiences and their emotions could lead to catastrophic behavior.[5]

Coste and her colleague in this work, Dr. Paul Raia, teach and recommend an alternative approach, habilitation therapy.[6] "The aim of habilitation therapy is not to restore people with a dementia such as Alzheimer's disease to what they once were," Raia writes, "but to maximize their functional independence and morale." This approach is "defined as a proactive environmental therapy characterized by creating and maintaining positive emotions." Raia identifies communication as the most critical area for eliciting positive emotions.[7]

Continuing my reading in *Learning to Speak Alzheimer's*, I was intrigued to learn how the earlier scene might have unfolded with a staff member trained in the habilitation model of communicating.

When Mary expressed her wish to see her mother, the nursing aide said, simply, "Tell me about her."

"She's a great cook," Mary said.

"What does she make that you especially like?"

"Oh, her pies are the best. I can never match 'em. Oh, dear, now I'm getting hungry."

Claire took Mary's hand and guided her toward the dining room. "Me, too," she said. "You have a cup of coffee while I go get your friend Pat—we'll be right back."

Dignity intact, free from medical or chemical restraint, Mary sat back with her coffee and awaited her friend's arrival. Thoughts of her mother faded, replaced by the positive experience of Claire's smiling face and extended hand.[8]

Somewhere over Michigan while reading this revised scene, it was as if a lightbulb appeared over my head. "Oh my God!" I heard myself exclaim out loud, "This woman is doing improv!" This was a moment of exceptional awareness, and I was thrilled to discover a way for communicating and connecting with Mom that was already familiar to me, meeting her in her improvised reality. I could do that!

I wondered if the author realized that she had described a beautifully crafted improv scene. Probably not, I concluded. It's more likely that Coste is a natural yes-sayer to the twists and turns of life. Acknowledging and accepting the uncontrollable changes perpetuated by her husband's dementia, she recognized that she had to "deal with the reality of today." "I vowed," she writes, "to learn to live with this person who was inhabiting the body of the man I cherished. I had to detach myself emotionally from the man my husband used to be and live now with the man he had become."[9]

Coste recommends that caregivers meet persons with Alzheimer's in their current place or time, in their world—wherever, whenever, whatever—that might be, and find joy with them there.[10] She encourages caregivers to be ready for anything to happen, therefore being alert and more able to respond appropriately to emotions that are being expressed beneath failing words. Describing her own attitudes toward her husband and her interactions with him, she models for caregivers how to be *willing*. Coste didn't instigate conflict, but she welcomed every conflict as an opportunity to ease her husband's suffering and to return from discord to peace.

Through my own clumsy efforts at improvising, I had learned that being ready for anything to happen and being willing to accept anything is easier said than done, especially if a person is naturally inclined to be a no-sayer, as I was at the time. From improvisation teacher Keith Johnstone, I learned more about this attitude and felt encouraged: "There are far more 'No' sayers around than 'Yes' sayers," according to Johnstone. And for good reason, in my opinion. "Those who say 'No' are rewarded by the safety they attain [whereas] those who say 'Yes' are rewarded by the adventures they have."[11]

As an Alzheimer's family caregiver, how I wanted to follow a safe path. But I learned from Coste that, for persons with the disease as well as for engaged caregivers, Alzheimer's is all about adventure. It's all about yes. Fortunately, Johnstone encouraged me by saying no-sayers can be trained to behave like yes-sayers.

According to Richard Rohr, all of life is a yes-saying training camp. He claims that the first half of life, "when we are naturally and rightly preoccupied with establishing our identity —climbing, achieving, and performing, defines itself by 'No.'" We are staying safe. The second half of life takes us on a "further journey," he writes, "one that involves challenges, mistakes, loss of control, broader horizons and necessary suffering that actually shocks us out of our comfort zone." This further journey is defined by "Yes!"[12]

Johnstone's version of saying yes from the perspective of improvisation sounds enticing: "adventure." Rohr's version of saying yes, from the perspective of the spiritual journey, sounds challenging: "shocked out of our comfort zone." From the perspective of a recovering no-sayer, I learned that engagement with both versions requires intention, practice, and the courage to unconditionally choose to say "Yes!" In addition, I learned that saying yes to the challenges, mistakes, loss of control, broader horizons, and necessary suffering that constitute the adventure of Alzheimer's disease also requires compassion, love, and an openness to being transformed.

My efforts to heal from my failed relationship had led me to the broader horizons of improvisation and helped me to see my life pattern of resistance. Prior to this time, I used will, skill, and effort, trying to make situations fit my preferences when I didn't like or want what was happening. This endeavor was exhausting and usually futile.

When this approach is implemented in an improvised scene, it's called "blocking the offer." This is in the realm of no-saying. Scared improvisers are seeking safety, leading inevitably to a very bad scene. My own fear and resistance became crystal clear during a class scene when my partner said, "I've dropped my contact lens on the floor." I blocked this offer and negated her reality when I said, "Oh no. It's probably still in your eye. Let me look." When I moved closer to have a look, I might have stepped on her contact, creating all kinds of conflict. My no-saying impulse was so strong that, even in a class during a theater game, I couldn't accept the offer my partner had extended, that she dropped her contact lens. I could have made the obvious response and said, "Yikes? Contact on the floor! I'm afraid to move." Then my partner would have felt validated, and an interesting scene might have evolved. What happened instead was conflict. "No," she said as she pushed me away. "I dropped it." This was *her* reality.

Improvisation, I learned, is not about being clever or original. It's about being obvious.[13] It's about accepting the offer that has been extended by your scene partner, considering it valid, and then saying or doing the next logical thing. To do improv well, we need to be willing to say yes—to accept what's happening and what's said as true and valid—even when our scene partner offers a new or surprising direction. As improv coach Katie Goodman explains, our willing yes is "not from a complacent or docile position but from a bouncy 'bring it on' space."[14] From this bouncy place, there is endless freedom and possibility.

The opportunity for me to practice saying a bouncy yes in the context of Alzheimer's arose during my first day alone with Mom. Fortunately, awareness about what was happening dawned on me, and thankfully, inspiration came from somewhere. Using the improv techniques I had been studying, I facilitated a turning point that took me onto the road of adventure and discovery.

Mom and I were sitting at the dining room table playing cribbage, a game we had enjoyed playing together for more than forty years. In fact, the story went around our neighborhood that I had learned to count 15-2, 15-4, 15-6 before I learned to count 1-2-3. The game was going along quite well. Mom was playing in a way that didn't reveal her diminishing cognitive abilities. She was winning as usual, but she must have thought I was getting too close for comfort. In the middle of a hand, she stopped playing and said, "You're very good at this game."

"Well, thank you," I replied.

"Who taught you how to play?" Mom asked.

This question caught me completely by surprise. Mom had taught me to play, so I decided to remind her.

"You did," I told her.

"No, I didn't."

Doesn't she remember? I thought. "Yes, you did," I said.

"No, I didn't."

How could she not remember? "YES, you did," I said emphatically, thinking that my mighty resistance would somehow help her to remember and admit her error.

"No, I didn't!" Mom resisted my resistance with even greater emphasis, becoming visibly agitated.

We continued like this for several seconds: "Yes, you did." "No, I didn't." As Mom became more and more agitated, I felt more and more anxious. Finally, in an attempt to distract her from our differing recollections, I tried a technique I had heard about, redirecting.

"It's your play," I said, trying to return her attention to the game.

It worked! She was redirected, and the game continued. I was relieved, but only briefly. A few minutes later, seeming to remember the earlier conversation, Mom said, "No, really, who taught you how to play?"

I also remembered our agitated discussion and didn't want to repeat it. Calling upon my improv training, I spoke the truth, but a little differently.

"No, really, who taught you how to play?" Mom asked again.

"My mother did," I replied.

"Oh," Mom said with surprise in her voice. "I didn't know that Aunt Stella knew how to play cribbage."

Aunt Stella! My mother? What?

A few heartbeats later, I realized that something in Mom's diminishing brain was telling her that I was her cousin, Alice. I was sitting just two feet away from her, and she didn't recognize me, her daughter. What was going on? I was shocked but decided to follow Coste's suggestion. I put myself into Mom's world at this moment—wherever that was, I had no idea. But I said, "Yes, my mother was a very good cribbage player."

"And she was a very good cook too," Mom added with certainty.

I had never met Mom's aunt Stella, but I remembered the story about cooking from *Learning to Speak Alzheimer's*, so I borrowed the line.

"What did Aunt Stella make that you liked best?"

"Kneffles!" Mom replied, smiling with enthusiasm.

For a while, we talked about Aunt Stella's cooking and how to make kneffles (German noodles). Then the game joyfully continued. Mom won, of course!

Family members often feel hurt and frustrated when loved ones with Alzheimer's don't remember our names, or if and how we're related. In these instances the losses of Alzheimer's are heightened, and the pain feels so heavy it can become almost unbearable. Through the lens of improvisation, however, families might come to understand that recognizing and playing the roles we've been cast into—instead of demanding to be ourselves—may enhance our connections with our loved ones. We can create joyful, healing moments instead of hurtful, heartbreaking ones.

In the earlier stages, persons with Alzheimer's are aware that they are forgetting important things and people. Correcting them about our names and relationships could feel demeaning and humiliating to them. Or as I discovered, correcting them could aggravate them because they will relentlessly perceive us to be wrong. There is a subtle point to consider, however. In the early stage, reminding them who we are might actually be helpful. For example, when coming into the room, it can be a good idea to make eye contact and say, "Hi, Mom, it's Jade, your daughter." This is a reminder, not a correction, and is different from saying, "No, Mom. I'm not Alice, your cousin. Don't you know me? It's me, Jade, your daughter."[15]

Under completely different circumstances, when I was younger, I would feel slighted and very hurt when Mom called me by my sibling's name. So I was surprised not to feel slighted during the confused and confusing conversation that erupted during the cribbage game. Seemingly, my excitement overcame any potential upset over not being recognized. In a situation simmering with conflict and hurt feelings, I had figured out something to say that resulted in a touching and happy outcome. A true connection had taken place. Being cast as Alice didn't cause emotional upset because I instinctively knew, in that moment and through the rest of Mom's life with Alzheimer's, that she was doing her best. She looked at me and saw her beloved Alice. I didn't understand *how* this was possible, but I did understand that it *was* possible.

Throughout our time together, Mom seamlessly moved in and out of current reality without any warning. One minute I was her daughter; the next, I was someone else.

For Valentine's Day that year, I had sent Mom an amethyst bracelet handmade for her by an artist friend of mine. My sibling told me that it had broken and they had thrown it away. Imagine my surprise when, one day, Mom and I were looking for her earrings and I came across the bracelet in her jewelry box. Only the clasp was broken.

"Look, Mom," I said, "here's the bracelet I sent you. The clasp is broken, but all the pieces are here. I'll take it all back to Maine with me, and I'll ask the artist to fix it for you."

I picked up the bracelet, and Mom looked very worried. "You can't take that," she said. "My daughter gave that to me."

Who she thought I was at this time wasn't clear. Nor was it clear exactly when she had shifted out of current reality and lost her ability to recognize me. But still, sweet tears welled up in my eyes as I realized that six months after she had received this gift, she remembered that it had come from me.

"OK," I said. "I won't take it with me. But what if we mail it to your daughter and ask her to have it fixed."

"That would be good," Mom replied, her worried expression fading. "It's pretty. I'd like to wear it."

"Let's go to the store and get a padded envelope, and then we can go to the post office and mail it."

Mom said, "OK."

And so we did. I mailed the bracelet to myself. Mission accomplished. Mom's beliefs, wishes, and current reality were honored, and I relive this charming experience of connection every time I wear her bracelet.

At other times, there were people in Mom's world to whom I had no access. To stay grounded during this family visit, one morning I went to an Alanon meeting. Still unaware at the time about the perils of leaving her alone, I thought she would be fine. When I came home, she was standing in the middle of the den with a mystified look on her face.

"Hi, Mom," I said tentatively, gently touching her shoulder.

"Is everything all right?"

"There was a man here," she said. "He came to the door and told me that my father said he could spend the night here. I don't know where he should sleep."

"Well," I replied, pausing to accept this as valid and to consider the next logical thing to say. "Let's look at the possibilities." We then walked through the house and discussed various options. When we got to the top of the basement steps, Mom said, "I told him he couldn't sleep down there." (It was my sibling's room.) We evaluated other options and finally decided that our guest could sleep on the sofa bed in the living room. A gracious hostess, Mom collected sheets and blankets and a pillow, which she gently laid on the sofa. I suggested we wait to make up the bed until later. After Mom went to bed that night, I put everything away.

The next afternoon, Mom came to me with a man's white shirt, nicely ironed and on a hanger.

"That man must have left this shirt behind," she said.

I had no idea who owned this shirt, but I said, "I'm sure he'll be back for it. Let's hang it in the closet so it doesn't get wrinkled." This we did, and that was the last I heard about my grandfather's mysterious friend.

My expectations of Mom began to shift into the realm of realism according to Alzheimer's, and I began to accept that what's happening is what's happening. Making this important shift planted another seed for the healing of our relationship as well as for developing skills for effective Alzheimer's caregiving.

During those weeks with Mom, I welcomed and enjoyed daily opportunities to meet her in her reality and learn more about her world. I practiced recognizing and playing my role, and when I was successful, Mom's behavior didn't remotely resemble what my sibling had described—thankfully.

Given the expectations my sibling and the Alzheimer's

Association website had established for me, Mom continually surprised me. Much to my relief, the nonalcoholic beer I gave her was received as an acceptable substitute for the real thing, and she guzzled it with gusto! She even took all of her pills cooperatively.

Not as advertised, Mom's appetite was ravenous. However, her quirky preference that we eat the same things had survived Alzheimer's, and I worried because our diets were vastly different: meat and potatoes versus macrobiotic vegan. When I tried to make a hamburger for Mom as an alternative to the chickpea burger I was making for myself, she adamantly refused. Although I knew she'd like the hamburger better, I followed her lead, and we both ate chickpea burgers that night. Throughout my visit, Mom adapted to my vegetarian diet, pronouncing everything I made for her "delicious." As long as we had the exact same food on our plates, she was happy.

There were some episodes, though, where I missed my cue, and a meaningful yes was either delayed or altogether absent. These experiences helped me to understand more about the moods, behaviors, and challenges my sibling and other caregivers described.

Mom's doctor had prescribed vitamin B-12 because a deficiency can increase memory disorders. We had gone to the kind of funky, kind of dingy health food store in town to buy ingredients for my recipes. On the shelf, I saw B-12, showed Mom, and headed to the checkout with the bottle. Her face instantly red and her eyes flaring with anger, Mom snatched the bottle from my hand. Through clenched teeth she said, "I'm not getting this."

The Mom I knew was all about appearances, so I was shocked by her angry reaction in a public place. Not welcoming a confusing scene escalating in the store, I didn't try to convince her that the doctor wanted her to take this. I timidly said, "OK," and put the bottle back on the shelf. We bought our food and left the store.

Although I was rattled by Mom's public anger, I was equally curious about what had happened. As soon as I regained my composure, I was able to shift into improv mode and logically inquire about Mom's world. "Why didn't you want the B-12? Your doctor thinks it might be helpful for you. He prescribed it."

"Well," Mom said, her posture huffy and her tone arrogant, "I'm not getting it there. I want to get it at Hartig's (her drugstore)."

Ohhhh. It was the funky, dingy store she was resisting! It never would have occurred to me that this was the source of her resistance. We went to Hartig's, bought the B-12 and went home. Mom took it right away.

I was grateful that my curiosity carried me back into Mom's moment where I was able to meet her and to learn more about her reasons for resisting. I assumed that people with Alzheimer's couldn't think or decide—and that we needed to think and decide for them. I learned from Mom that this presumption could make people with Alzheimer's justifiably angry. Without this moment of connection, I might have reported Mom to her doctor as being angry, uncooperative, and refusing her prescribed medications. The result for her could have been weeks of being out of it from the antipsychotic medication the doctor was prescribing to make her more cooperative. This medication was essentially taking away her will.

Years later, I learned from the work of Tom Kitwood and Kathleen Bredin that assertive behavior from a person with Alzheimer's, which is usually in the form of dissent, is a sign of well-being, and can be observed even into the later stages of the disease process.[16] By meeting Mom in her moment of resistance instead of trying to convince her to buy the vitamins, I learned something about the status of her mental abilities, her preferences, and her desire to be heard and taken seriously. I also learned something about the importance of being respectful in the context of cognitive decline, and not assuming that I always knew—more clearly than Mom did—what she wanted or was thinking, or what was best for her.

One afternoon, we were preparing dinner together. Mom's attention to detail and her ability to concentrate on a task were astounding, making her the absolute best assistant cook. Initiating what I thought was idle conversation, I asked her if she liked her primary care doctor. (We had an appointment to see him in a few days.)

"No, I don't," she vehemently replied.

"Really? Why not?" I was surprised by her clarity.

"Because he always speaks to the other adult in the room." Again, I was surprised by her clarity.

Mom still knew that she was a person in the room and should be directly spoken to by her doctor. And she knew what was in her heart and her mind and could still communicate about this—if asked. I had to learn how to draw her out, then how to listen and hear her. After I became Mom's guardian and had the authority to do so, I changed her doctor.

There was another poignant learning time that helped me to understand my sibling's description of Mom as angry, uncooperative, and combative. At this moment of learning, I felt especially helpless, and "Yes" remained unspoken.

When Mom and I met with her neurologist, he suggested that she attend an adult day center in order to maintain her verbal skills through practice and to uplift her emotional state through socialization. After making arrangements with a social worker from the Alzheimer's Association to accompany us to the local centers for tours, I told Mom about the plan. She adamantly refused to go, accusing me of coming to Iowa to "garage" her away. As I rationally refuted this, explaining that the neurologist thought it would be beneficial, Mom became frustrated and upset because I wasn't hearing her, and she slapped my forearm. This ended the scene instantly. Startled and upset, I started to cry. Mom fled the house by the side door and stomped furiously through her backyard. As if restrained by an invisible fence, she stopped right at the edge of her yard and looked out over the expanse of neighboring backyards. She stood there for a long time, looking—feeling bewildered and frightened, I assumed but didn't know for sure. Watching her from inside the house, ensuring that she was safe, my heart recognized her diminishing independence and just knew how much she hated that. Without effort or conscious thought, my tears of surprise and hurt transformed to tears of compassion.

Although I didn't know what to do next, I didn't want to leave Mom alone. As soon as I felt calm enough, I took some birdseed outside and stood next to her. I took her hand and said, "Here's your birdseed, Mom. Let's feed your birds." This was Mom's favorite activity. She took the seed from me and fed her birds. The adult day center was not mentioned again.

My study of Alzheimer's on the plane had informed me that Mom's behavior did not include an intention to be uncooperative or willful. She was trying to preserve her dignity and to communicate her needs and desires, using her remaining, although limited, cognitive abilities. She was marching to her own tune. With the help of improvisation, I was able to get into step with her, and with only a few glitches, our time together went very well. We became close and compatible companions.

In her own way, Mom was able to tell me that my efforts to learn about Alzheimer's, my attempts to communicate creatively, my compassionate attention, and my curiosity had made an impression on her. The day before I was leaving to return to Maine, Mom looked up at me from her chair in the living room and said, "Will you stay and take care of me? You're so kind to me."

To my recollection, my fiercely independent, highly competent mother had never before asked me—or anyone—for help. So unexpected and stunning was this moment that it remains etched in my memory even now. The experience of hearing this request from Mom and seeing the sincere pleading in her eyes opened my heart. Although I quietly explained to her that I would do my best to return and be her "guardian angel," my heart shouted out, "Yes!"

Waiting and Preparing

My own dawning awareness of Mom's obvious decline awakened the mother lion within me. My natural instincts toward Mom became sweetly tender and fiercely protective. During her early years with the disease, I was powerless to care for her in any meaningful way because my sibling had complete control. As is often the case for out-of-town family members, my input was not welcome, and although it was difficult for me, I had to accept this. After Mom noticed my kindness, however, and asked me to stay and take care of her, I made a herculean attempt to become her legal guardian. Unfortunately, the Iowa courts were not favorable toward out-of-state relatives seeking guardianship at that time. Although I was willing to move to Iowa if granted guardianship, I had little hope of success. My sibling was already living with Mom.

Accepting that family and legal circumstances beyond my control would allow me to care about Mom only from a distance was pure anguish for me. One day, in the midst of my despair, the closing lines from Mary Oliver's poem "The Journey" drifted into my consciousness. I was reminded that the only life I could save was my own. As I wept, I felt held and consoled by this poem.

Although I felt truly overwhelmed by my helplessness, I knew that Oliver's words were true. I couldn't "save" Mom. Not now anyway. Still, I didn't like feeling so disempowered. Soon after returning home to Maine, I tried to defeat my helplessness by seeking out additional legal opinions. One Iowa lawyer who was particularly insightful and helpful reviewed the case, counseled me in important ways, and then offered the frustrating advice to "sit tight until something significant happens." This advice was hard to take, partly because I was standing at a crossroad in my own life, ready to leave Maine. It would have been perfect timing for me to move to Iowa. I learned through this experience, however, that sometimes it's important to just wait.

What some could interpret as caregivers doing nothing might actually be a manifestation of wisdom, spiritual maturity, and active waiting. In the world of Alzheimer's, sometimes the most prudent action is to pause patiently in awareness and readiness for life and circumstances to unfold. When caregivers are caught in these complex situations of family and illness, our embrace of this process and our response at the appropriate time will make all the difference in the lives of our loved ones.

Saving the only life I could save—my own—was all I could do at the time. I didn't know it then, but accepting my limitations and focusing on my own health and well-being would benefit both Mom and me in the future. Much later, I realized that maintaining good self-care for myself throughout Mom's journey through Alzheimer's gave me a strong foundation for building a better quality of life for her. At the time, however, I felt that I had failed Mom. Not being able to fulfill her request—to stay with her and to care for her kindly—remains one of my life's greatest regrets.

Since caring for and about Mom from a distance was my only option, I decided to walk with her by learning more about Alzheimer's and the family dynamics associated with Alzheimer's care. With this goal in mind, I contacted a psychiatrist in the Portland area, Dr. William Berlingieri. He had been the medical director of a nursing home system in Massachusetts for many years and had evaluated thousands of persons with Alzheimer's and related disorders. When I told him about discovering the improvisation-Alzheimer's connection, he was overjoyed. To my surprise, he said that many years earlier he had tried to hire improvisers from ImprovBoston and Improv Asylum[17] to come to his nursing homes. He wanted them to teach his staff how to communicate effectively with persons with dementia using improv techniques. Unfortunately, his board of directors, administrators, and nurses resisted this approach. There had been controversy in the field. Any creative ways of communicating with persons with memory loss, particularly those that veered away from reality orientation, were considered by some to be undignified. There was especially prickly resistance, bordering on outrage, if creative communication involved any kind of fantasy interaction that could be interpreted as lying.

To counter concerns like this, which are prevalent among Alzheimer's families and caregivers, and to relieve creative, yes-saying caregivers of guilt they might harbor about lying, Paul Raia, explains, "These are not lies, these are what I call 'therapeutic fiblettes'—inroads into the patient's reality. It is only if we become comfortable and creative in the use of the fiblettes that we become effective [caregivers]."[18] The world of improv teaches us to say the next logical thing when someone makes an offer. The next logical thing to say when persons with Alzheimer's speak from their improvisational reality may not seem true or logical in our world, but it will seem just right in their world. And the reality of their world is where we must and will meet them.

Dr. Berlingieri became a valued teacher as I explored ways to unravel and integrate the mystery of Alzheimer's into my life, to effectively communicate with Mom, and to understand how

Alzheimer's was stirring up dormant family dynamics. Through our many discussions, he shared his experience and wisdom and helped me begin to formulate a deeper understanding of how to be a compassionate and effective Alzheimer's caregiver.

Many people would like medical science to provide absolute guidelines about how to interact and communicate with persons with Alzheimer's. But Dr. Berlingieri helped me to understand that science doesn't consider the unique way every human being experiences life, especially when the brain is altered by disease and thought processes and behaviors become unpredictable. Therefore, the *phenomenology* of Alzheimer's—those qualities and practices that can be observed through our senses and intuition in the presence of those afflicted—is the most informative and reliable guide for creating satisfying interpersonal experiences when interacting with this population. Because of the decline of cognition and capacity in persons with Alzheimer's, and their ever-changing, ever-increasing needs, caregivers' observation skills are crucial to the well-being of those afflicted.

We have to accept that, as the disease process relentlessly marches on, persons with Alzheimer's will not be the most reliable reporters of what is happening to them. Declining verbal abilities will make it difficult for them to report side effects of medications, to be specific about pain, or to clearly express their wants and needs. Facial expressions, body language, and sounds are the caregivers' guides, and being attentive in new ways becomes a necessity. Persons with Alzheimer's won't remember if they've eaten meals or taken medication. Caregiving therefore requires vigilance in recognizing and responding to what needs to be done for them. Doing so without negating their remaining autonomy by imposing unnecessary, demeaning assistance becomes the challenge. Regular schedules and structure are both helpful tools for caregivers seeking cooperation and beneficial for persons with Alzheimer's. Bodies instinctively and readily adapt to routines. Adopting a specific, consistent time for medication, a nap, a walk, or meals will avert stress and conflict because it will feel right to the person with Alzheimer's when a caregiver says, "It's time." Upon receiving the diagnosis of this degenerative terminal illness, persons with Alzheimer's may exhibit distress over the diagnosis and having to cope with the changes they experience. At this time, medical and psychiatric interventions for anxiety, depression, and insomnia, including medications, may be useful. As the disease progresses, however, mind and emotion-altering medicine will not help or change them, especially in the later stages. Persons with Alzheimer's have a way of organizing and responding to the information they have in their brains at any given time, and we can't change them. This is a challenge for our society in general because we are accustomed to a prescriptive response to illness. Since we do not, at this time, have medicines to cure or delay Alzheimer's, our challenges are the following:

- to accept the current prognosis of the illness and its relentless progression
- to move away from our prescriptive inclinations to medicate symptoms and seek alternative interventions
- to commit ourselves to learn about and understand what is happening for persons with Alzheimer's, so we can communicate, connect, and care effectively

Over all, we caregivers need to overcome our resistance to accepting the illness, change the ways we meet the realities of persons with Alzheimer's, and embrace their moments. We regularly engage in fantasy play with children without hesitation or guilt. Engaging with persons with Alzheimer's in their world is a similar activity. It's not about lying; it's about imagination, connection, respect, and enjoyment. Most importantly, we want persons with Alzheimer's to feel that they have been heard and that their concerns are being taken seriously.

Dr. Berlingieri brought to my attention one aspect of Alzheimer's that must be accepted: It is impossible to reach consensus reality with persons who have lost the ability to gather and analyze new data or to shift their thinking at will. "Consensus reality" was a new concept for me, and I wasn't exactly sure how it related to my interactions with Mom or the differences in our perceptions and recollections. As I wondered more about this concept, I remembered a story about an elephant and blind men that I had first heard as a child. This ancient parable from the Jain religious tradition of India explained to me what consensus reality means in relationship to persons with Alzheimer's: Maybe they have their reasons for doing and saying what they're doing and saying.

Once upon a time, there lived six blind men in a village. One day the villagers told them, "Hey, there is an elephant in the village today." The blind men had no idea what an elephant was, but they decided, "Even though we would not be able to see it, let us go and feel it anyway." All of them went to where the elephant was, and every one of them touched the elephant.

"Hey, the elephant is like a tree," said the first man, who touched his leg.

"Oh, no! It is like a rope," said the second man, who touched the tail.

"Oh, no! It is like a snake," said the third man, who touched the trunk of the elephant.

"It is like a big hand fan," said the fourth man, who touched the ear of the elephant.

"It is like a huge wall," said the fifth man, who touched the belly of the elephant.

"It is like a spear," said the sixth man, who touched the tusk of the elephant.

They began to argue about the elephant, every one

of them insisting that he was right. It looked like they were getting agitated. A wise man was passing by and he saw this.

He stopped and asked them, "What is the matter?"

They said, "We cannot agree to what the elephant is like." Each one of them told what he thought the elephant was like.

The wise man calmly explained to them, "All of you are right. The reason every one of you is telling it differently is because each of you touched a different part of the elephant. Actually, the elephant has all the features you describe."

"Oh!" everyone said.

There was no more fighting. They felt happy that all of them were right.

The moral of the story in the Jain tradition is that there may be some truth in what someone says. Sometimes we can see that truth and sometimes not. Others may have a different perspective with which we may not agree, but rather than arguing, like the blind men, we should say, "Maybe you have your reasons." This way we don't get in arguments. This allows us to live in harmony with the people of different thinking. [19]

In the story, each blind man's position about the elephant is valid because it comes from empirical experience, which is impossible to challenge. When persons with Alzheimer's share their "different thinking" with us, we often can't see what they're seeing. And from their perspective, they can't see what we're seeing. Even though it's not easy to surrender our own reality, that's exactly what we need to do. Trying to convince persons with Alzheimer's that we're right or trying to persuade them to do what we want them to do is a sure recipe for conflict—and possibly disaster. Therefore, we need to give them opportunities to show us their realities so we can meet them there. I discovered that this requires patience, attention, open-mindedness, and a willingness to be surprised.

When Leslie's father Arnold moved into an assisted-living facility, he created quite a stir. He refused to get out of bed in the morning and after naps, explaining that there were things on the floor, and he didn't want to step on them. There was nothing on the floor, but he insisted there was. Every morning and at other times during the day, there was a fight to get him out of bed, which generated distress for Arnold and aides alike.

Observing this situation, most would conclude that Arnold was hallucinating. But his concerned and aware daughter noticed that there was a section of wood paneling on the wall that resembled the flooring material. On this wood paneling hung a clock and a thermostat, "things" her father could see while lying in his bed. Leslie enlisted the assistance of a nurse to cover the wood wall paneling with fabric. This simple intervention erased Arnold's concern about the things on the floor. Now he gets up every day without worry or resistance. He wasn't hallucinating after all. Indeed, he had his reasons.

While I was waiting for something significant to happen that would open the door for me to be an active participant in Mom's care, I also continued to explore the intersection of Alzheimer's disease and improvisation. Will Luera, artistic director of ImprovBoston, had come to Maine to teach classes for my improvisation practice group. Impressed by Luera's interpersonal sensitivity as well as his talent, I contacted him to explore his interest in helping me develop a workshop for communicating with persons with Alzheimer's using improvisation. Previously, I had mentioned that I was discovering spiritual components in improvisation, and he was fascinated. Now I hoped he would help me incorporate these spiritual components for healing into the creation of an improv workshop for Alzheimer's caregivers.

The improv way of being in the world can open doors to spirituality. This awareness manifested into reality in the context of Alzheimer's caregiving when I was able to meet Mom in her world because, there, we both experienced healing.

Some of the spiritual elements I discovered while implementing improv techniques in Mom's presence are:

- meeting in true connection
- being present in *this* moment
- expanding awareness of myself and others
- increasing observation through the senses
- letting go of the need, and even the desire, to control
- letting go of the need to know what happens next
- accepting and surrendering to what is; saying yes to reality
- finding the gifts in every experience
- responding in a way that is supportive and promotes self-esteem and dignity
- acknowledging interdependence
- experiencing, embracing, and expressing joy moment by moment

When I described how the integration of the spiritual aspects I had experienced in the context of improv could provide healing for persons with Alzheimer's and their caregivers, Luera was intrigued. The potential of such a creative and purposeful application for the craft he loved inspired him. He immediately agreed to help with the workshop and was on the next train to Maine. We ate soup, walked by the ocean, and gave birth to the Healing Moments programs for persons with Alzheimer's and their families, friends, and caregivers.

Over the winter, the psychiatrist, the improviser, and the minister met several times, sharing our wisdom about Alzheimer's caregiving from our three different perspectives and areas of expertise. The building blocks from this unique collaboration became the foundation for caregiving techniques that would be life-changing for me, for Mom, and for others with dementia.

After completing my spiritual direction training in the spring of 2005, I left Maine and moved back to Boston. I wanted to pursue two programs of study that, to an objective observer, may have seemed completely unrelated: improvisation and a doctorate of ministry in faith, health, and spirituality. To me, these areas of interest had become inseparable.

During my first day of class at ImprovBoston, my teacher said something profound and unforgettable: "The first rule of improvisation is to make your scene partner look good." This rule eventually became my mantra for compassionate, effective Alzheimer's caregiving.

Then the significant something I had been waiting for happened. In September of 2006, my sibling moved Mom to a nursing home. Six months later, my sibling moved away. Over the next year, these actions caused me, literally, to emotionally and physically move back and forth across the threshold between Mom's world and my world. As Rumi's poem advises, I did not go back to sleep.

Into the Heart of Alzheimer's

A Refiner's Fire is not indiscriminate.
It is used to purify,
to burn away what is not needed
and to leave the precious gold and silver.
—inspired by Malachi 2:17–3:6

Relief was my initial reaction when I learned that Mom had moved to a nursing home. I no longer had to worry about her walking into traffic, drinking alcohol, missing meals, burning herself with hot water, falling and freezing, or cooking and setting herself on fire. She would be "safe." This move also opened the door for me to have more contact with Mom and to be more involved in her life and her care.

During my winter break from school, I went to Iowa for several days. Although nursing homes were not among my most desired settings, being reunited with Mom after two and a half years—no matter where—warmed my heart. I was delighted to notice some of Mom's remaining skills, which included recognizing me—I was still her "girl"—and reading her name. Every time we passed the door to her room, she paused and read her name aloud. Meeting Mom's social worker, advocate, and nurses helped me to understand her current life and needs. When it was time to return to Boston, it was hard to leave her.

My sibling's move out of town three months later muddied my relief. Mom was alone in a nursing home, "garaged" and abandoned. This had to be her worst nightmare. For me, however, it was no longer the perfect time to relocate to Iowa. I was happy being back in Boston after seven years in Maine. My doctor of ministry program, focusing on spirituality and spiritual direction for seminarians, was exactly the study I felt called to pursue. It was my life's work, I was sure.

At this juncture, my experience of going back and forth across the threshold of Mom's world of Alzheimer's in Iowa and my world of spiritual study in Boston seized my soul. I *had* to do something, and considered a variety of options. One possibility included relocating Mom to Massachusetts. Although I didn't have the legal authority at the time to move her, I investigated and toured nursing homes near my apartment. Another option was to rent small apartments in both Massachusetts and Iowa and be with Mom during school breaks. That summer, I went to Iowa for seven weeks to further explore the possibility of having dual residences.

After being with Mom, and after much going back and forth emotionally, I moved to Iowa in February 2008. When I made the decision, I thought I would need to discontinue my doctoral studies. The professors and school administrators, however, agreed to work with me from a distance. That first semester, an e-course called Ministry to the Elderly was offered. "Ah," I thought, "Since I'm going to be in a nursing home every day, this could be helpful."

Indeed it was! It also changed the whole course of my doctoral studies. This course opened the door for the practical integration of my academic interests in spirituality and my personal experiences with Alzheimer's. As I became engulfed by the refiner's fire of Alzheimer's care and learning, what I began to see emerging from the fire was indeed pure gold and shining silver.

Walking together, into the fire . . .

Healing When
There Is No Cure

One recent afternoon, I was having tea with my friend Janaan. A few years ago, her beloved husband Carl died after a long journey through an Alzheimer's-type dementia. Without question, Janaan and Carl were on the journey together, and she considered each day with him an opportunity for loving. As we shared stories about caring for Carl and Mom, Janaan said, "If I had it to do over, I would, gratefully. And," she added with endearing certainty, "I would do it better." "Oh," I thought, with tears in my eyes. "How I *wish* I could do it over. How I wish I could have known at the beginning of my caregiving journey with Mom what I knew at the end!" Given my rich learning and experience, I would have been an even better caregiver.

After many years of caring for his beloved wife Virginia, Cape Cod writer Elliot Stanley Goldman reached this conclusion: "Alzheimer's is not a doctor's disease. It belongs to caregivers—family, nurses, aides—who see the patient through the long affliction for which there is no cure and no clear guidelines for what to expect at any stage."[1]

Over a decade after Goldman wrote those words, his conclusion remains true. In fact, it has been true since in 1906, when German physician Alois Alzheimer dissected the brain of Auguste D., a deceased patient he had met five years earlier. During their first meetings, Auguste's observable symptoms included "unexplainable bursts of anger, and then a strange series of memory problems." A skilled diagnostician, Alzheimer followed systematic protocol with Auguste in an effort to exclude certain conditions and discover the cause of her symptoms. But after ruling out all known diseases as the possible cause of an illness that presented as a psychiatric disorder, Alzheimer was left with a mystery. Throughout her illness, Auguste remained hospitalized, experiencing a steady decline of her remaining capacities and receiving what would today be identified as palliative care. The treatment goals were to keep her safe, clean, and as comfortable as possible.[2]

Alzheimer's autopsy of Auguste's brain revealed "peculiar clumps" (now known as *plaques*) and "a tangled bundle of fibrils" (now known as *tangles*) never before observed by medical scientists.[3] Over a hundred years later, these menacing plaques and tangles may be the basis of an epidemic of startling proportions. Currently, it's estimated that approximately 5.2 million Americans of all ages have Alzheimer's disease,[4] the most common form of dementia. Looking into the future at this disease, the "number of people 65 and older with Alzheimer's is estimated to reach 7.1 million in 2025. . . . By 2050, the number of individuals aged 65 and older with Alzheimer's is projected to number between 13.8 million and 16 million."[5]

Anticipating this daunting public health emergency, most of us are counting on medical breakthroughs that will identify ways to prevent or more effectively treat the disease. Unfortunately, the breakthroughs have not yet happened. Notable as the sixth-leading cause of death across all ages in the United States,[6] Alzheimer's disease continues to vex the most brilliant scientific and medical minds. Millions of research dollars are devoted to this critical effort. Since we are all potentially at the mercy of this disease, particularly as we age, finding cause and cure, and identifying preventive methods are urgent priorities. As Alzheimer's researcher Zaven Khachaturian asserts, "We have to solve this problem, or it's going to overwhelm us. . . . the numbers are going to double every twenty years . . . the duration of the illness is going to get much longer. That's the really devastating part."[7]

"Human kind / Cannot bear very much reality," T. S. Eliot writes in his poem "Burnt Norton."[8] The reality of Alzheimer's we can't bear is that this incurable disease of epidemic proportions continues to evade identification of cause and cure, and carries a devastating prognosis for individuals, families, and society. Caregivers who are committed to enhancing the lives of persons with Alzheimer's, however, must begin to find ways to endure what many consider unendurable.

When Virginia Goldman was diagnosed with Alzheimer's in the early 1990s, her husband heard nothing optimistic from doctors. Accustomed to the medical approach of curing disease, he was not initially prepared for the surrender that Alzheimer's demands. He recognized the need to embrace the concept of palliative care and ensure Virginia's comfort, and then attend first and foremost to her quality of life. However, living in a culture focused on conquering illness, he found himself standing uncomfortably at the intersection of his faith in medicine and the truth of Alzheimer's.[9]

The truth of Alzheimer's is that there isn't much doctors following traditional prescriptive protocols *can* do. The disciplines of science and medicine, together, are trying to make a difference and show us the way through the mystery of Alzheimer's. However, beyond a few medications that may or may not delay progression of the disease, the most recommended treatment is still the palliative care that Auguste D. received a century ago: "providing basic comfort as patients wait to die."[10] This remains the most common approach when the medical field declares, "There is nothing more we can do."

While investigating nursing homes for Mom during the going back and forth phase, I stumbled upon beautifully stated wisdom about treating terminal illnesses on the website of Luther Manor, a nursing home in Dubuque supported by a consortium of Lutheran churches in the county:

> Cure may occur without healing; healing may occur without cure.
> Cure looks at what sort of disease a person has; healing looks at what sort of person has the disease.
> Cure seeks ultimately to conquer pain; healing seeks to transcend pain.
> Cure is taunted by suffering; healing is taught by suffering.

Prompted by these words to research the author of these thought-provoking comparisons, I discovered that Lutheran pastoral theologian Fred Reklau had recognized and documented many more contrasts between healing and cure.

> Cure may occur without healing; healing may occur without cure.
> Cure separates body from soul; healing embraces the soul.
> Cure isolates; healing incorporates.
> Cure combats illness; healing fosters wellness.
> Cure fosters function; healing fosters purpose.
> Cure alters what is; healing offers what might be.
> Cure is an act; healing is a process.
> Cure acts upon another; healing shares with a sister, a brother.

Cure manages; healing touches.

Cure avoids grief; healing assumes grief.

Cure encounters mystery as a challenge for understanding; healing encounters mystery as a ready channel for meaning.

Cure rejects death and views it as defeat; healing includes death among the blessed outcomes of care.[11]

These distinctions enlightened my thinking about what healing means in the context of Alzheimer's and incurable diseases, reminding me that *cure* is a medical term and *healing* is a spiritual term. To heal means to "make whole." This is the life work of our souls and is not dependent on our physical well-being. This interpretation of healing helped me to more fully appreciate the writing of Dr. Arthur Kleinman, psychiatrist and caregiver for his wife Joan. Personally aware of the harsh realities of this disease, Kleinman believes the most effective treatment that physicians—or any healing professionals or caregivers—can offer to persons with Alzheimer's and their families is "some kind of caregiving and hope for the future."[12]

During my journey into Alzheimer's, I realized the truth of Kleinman's words. Caregiving and hope *are* the cornerstones for healing—in the absence of cure, they are all that's possible.

Elliot Goldman and Arthur Kleinman, both primary Alzheimer's caregivers for their wives, conclude that those in our society who truly have "expert knowledge" about Alzheimer's and the potential to bring about healing are the "spouses, children, friends, and the professional companions, aides, and nurses who do the actual caregiving—meaning everything from driving, walking with, reading to, feeding, bathing, and just being there for people whose brain is no longer capable of letting them be independent."[13] Through their writing, these expert caregivers are guides in the wilderness. Goldman, writing about his personal experiences with Alzheimer's in the 1990s, was a caregiving pioneer. By documenting and sharing the challenges and heartbreaks of his and Virginia's lives, Goldman charted new territory. He opened the door, giving others permission to reveal the truth of this disease and to share their thoughts, feelings, fears, frustrations, and confusion. His words of solidarity remind us that we are not alone.

Goldman understood the helplessness of persons with Alzheimer's, describing it with exquisite accuracy. He alerted me about how important my role as caregiver would be: "The caregiver is the patient's mentor, her eyes, her voice, the experience she lives in."[14] Reading this for the first time, realizing the truth and the enormity of Goldman's statement, all I could do was take a really deep breath. Then I prayed for the courage to come close to every aspect of Alzheimer's, for the strength to stay with Mom until the end, and for the humility to ask for help.

When Alzheimer's caregivers arrive at the intersection of cure and healing and find that only the road to healing is open for passage, many of us are, as Goldman was, unprepared and resistant. By describing Alzheimer's caregiving as a "defining moral practice," Kleinman gives us permission to release our dependence on medical science and the demand for a cure and to fully engage in the process of healing. Sharing an ancient Chinese perspective, Kleinman writes, "We are not born fully human, but only become so as we cultivate ourselves and our relations with others." He reminds us that healing results from the practice of companioning people who are in great need. He considers companioning a "moral practice that makes caregivers, and at times even the care receivers, more present and thereby more fully human."[15]

Medical science seeks to cure *diseases*. Caregiving, from the relational foundation Kleinman discusses, seeks healing for *persons* afflicted with diseases. When we offer care in the context of relationship, this action leads to self-cultivation that, even as we experience our limits and failures, facilitates our growth.[16]

Claiming that caregiving completes our humanity, this modern physician echoes the teaching of sixteenth-century Christian mystic Teresa of Avila, who characterized mature spiritual development as the awareness of God within "coupled with total availability to our neighbor without."[17]

For caregivers who have matured in modern American culture, where cure is almost revered, a conscious and deliberate shift away from our dependence on this scientific standard is needed to wholeheartedly accept healing.[18] The specific shift required in the context of Alzheimer's care is to encourage persons with the disease, their families, professional and informal caregivers, medical practitioners, religious communities, and society in general to recognize and value the life of the emotions and the spirit as well as the capacity of the mind. We also need to embrace our bodies as they reveal to us our natural human instinct, which is to grow into death.

Minds as well as hearts need to open. A shift in thinking will allow everyone, including scientists, scholars, and physicians, to see the old data regarding Alzheimer's disease through a new lens. According to Benedictine nun Joan Chittister, this shift will bring into focus a new perspective and restore all the dimensions that make up a self. Seeing things differently and valuing things differently allows us to give "honor where honor has far too long been lacking."[19]

Honoring the process of diminishment for persons with Alzheimer's over the futile effort to cure them reflects a worldview and attitude grounded in feminist teachings. Although there are more women in the world of caregiving, being female isn't necessary to manifest this different view and attitude. As Chittister writes, "It's . . . those qualities in both women and men that make feeling, compassion, heart, and service as important as reason, strength, law, and power."[20]

Kleinman, for example, believes that Alzheimer's caregiving based in relationship and moral acts comes before—and goes

beyond—mind-driven modern medicine.[21] Accordingly, Kleinman did not develop his compassionate way of seeing and acting in regard to Alzheimer's care in the classroom or the clinic.
There he learned about cure. He developed his compassionate
view in relationship, the heartbeat of healing. In his new life,
which consisted of daily care for Joan, Kleinman "learned to be
a caregiver by doing it." He writes, "I had to do it. It was there
to do." He adds a universal truth: "I think this is how most people learn to be caregivers for people who are elderly, disabled,
or chronically or terminally ill. But of course this is also how
parents, especially mothers, learn to care for children."[22]

Alzheimer's caregiving took Kleinman to the depths of his
being, where he discovered what all caregivers come to know,
that this is *not* easy:

> Caregiving consumes time, energy, and financial
> resources. It sucks out strength and determination. . . .
> It can amplify anguish and desperation. It can divide
> the self. It can bring out family conflicts. . . . It is also far
> more complex, uncertain, and unbounded than profes-
> sional medical and nursing models suggest.[23]
>
> Meeting these challenges unquestionably requires
> courage, commitment, and practice.

Resistance to—and possibly rejection of —efforts to care can
pose obstacles. Infants and toddlers, which persons with
Alzheimer's eventually come to resemble, are naturally receptive to the reciprocal practice of caregiving and care-receiving.
Unfortunately, persons with declining cognitive capacities, who
most need to practice receiving care and love, are often inclined
to resist their new roles as care receivers for as long as possible.
Their resistance is a by-product of a culture that places value
on productivity, autonomy, and independence. Needing and
receiving help is often interpreted as failure.

At a conference for Alzheimer's caregivers, I met Olivia Hoblitzelle. She shared with us heart-opening vignettes of companioning her husband through Alzheimer's. Hob Hoblitzelle's greatest fear related to his disease was "of being a nuisance." A devout and practicing Buddhist, Hob discussed his fear with his wise teacher Jim, whose reply reminds us that care receiving is another opportunity to consider life's challenges as lessons in becoming more fully human. "If you feel like you're being a nuisance, Hob, then you're going to have to learn to live with those feelings, too: letting people care for you, learning to receive. Consider all this a spiritual discipline!"[24]

There will come a time in the progression of Alzheimer's disease when the afflicted ones will lose their capacity to resist being given care. Should they live long enough to reach the end stages of the disease, this population will become completely helpless and then dependent upon and receptive to caregivers for their survival.[25] They will essentially regress to infancy and will then be among the most vulnerable members of our society.

Kleinman compares caregiving for someone with Alzheimer's to parenting, particularly mothering.[26] With this comparison, he ushers us onto holy ground. Adult children who are caregivers will especially recognize this role reversal with their parents who have Alzheimer's. If adult children choose to accept this new role, they will soon come to understand that the disease is calling them to transform their love and commitment into active caring. Like parents, they are called to take responsibility for the well-being and fulfillment of someone else.

In our culture, we most often take our model of love from romance. Theologian Sam Keen argues that, by stressing desire and excitement rather than "responsibility and care-giving" as the "central ingredients" of love," we create "immense confusion about the relationship between love and care." When this happens, "we tend to think of care-giving as a burden that, unfortunately, comes with long-term commitments."[27]

I have long believed that the deepest longing of every human soul is to love and be loved; that in loving and being loved we find meaning, purpose, and fulfillment in this life. Alzheimer's disease does not extinguish this longing.

Influenced by ancient and modern spiritual teachings, Keen and I are in agreement on this point: "Much of the meaning of our lives is created by tending, meeting, and taking responsibility for the well-being of others."[28] Keen warns us, however, that it's easy, and quite common, to dismiss this idea. "After all," he writes, "news of most any day suggests that what makes the world go round is not love, but fear, greed, competition, cruelty, and the will to power." As Erich Fromm told readers over fifty years ago in *The Art of Loving*, our culture has not encouraged us to explore the depths of loving, which includes care for the vulnerable among us. From the perspective of caring for the millions of vulnerable persons with Alzheimer's, it's disheartening to realize that not much social progress has been made toward the blossoming of love since then. Fromm writes, "In spite of the deep-seated craving for love, almost everything else is considered to be more important than love: success, prestige, money, power—almost all our energy is used for the learning of how to achieve these aims, and almost none to learn the art of loving."[29] From this perspective, our choices as caregivers—to move, to change our lives, to go to nursing homes every day and visit loved ones who don't remember us, to value the lives of persons with cognitive decline through fierce advocacy—are often met with confusion, skepticism, and even criticism by others.

However, the sacred importance of caregiving relationships has been a part of human consciousness since ancient times. According to Roman mythology, caregiving has the capacity to shape a being:

Once when Care was crossing a river, she saw some clay. Thoughtfully, she took a piece of the clay and began to shape it.

While she was meditating on what she had made, Jupiter, king of the Gods, came by. Care asked him to give her creation spirit, and this he gladly did. But when Care wanted her name to be bestowed upon it, Jupiter forbade this, and demanded that it be given his name instead.

While Care and Jupiter were arguing, Earth joined the dispute. Since Earth had furnished the clay from part of her own body, she expressed the desire for her own name to be conferred on the creature.

They decided to ask Saturn, the God of Time, to be their arbiter. Saturn made the following decision, which all believed to be a just one: "There is a dispute among you as to this creature's name. Let it be called homo-sapien for it is made out of humus—earth. Since you, Jupiter, have given its spirit, you shall receive that spirit at its death. Since you, Earth, have given its body, you shall receive its body. But most importantly, since Care first shaped this creature, she shall possess it as long as it lives."[30]

Devoted Alzheimer's caregivers are resurrecting this sacred understanding of care because we have experienced its relationship to the other elements of love. Through our practice of caregiving, many Alzheimer's caregivers have realized that the sacrifices demanded of us are making our lives richer with meaning, satisfaction, and expressions of true love than romance or sentimentality ever could.[31]

Arthur Kleinman touched my heart deeply with his words about caregiving and love:

The all-absorbing love I had for my wife and she for me, had more than sustained me and her through those uncertain years of building our professional lives, a family, and our own world. That fierce and joyful love had animated those years, now gone forever, with a golden hue that expressed a shared sensibility of things being right and good and beautiful. During the terrible years of Joan's descent through neurodegeneration to blindness, dementia, paralysis, and a slow death, love had made it possible to endure the unendurable; it motivated my caregiving and her care-receiving.[32]

Love can make it all possible.

I soon discovered that Kleinman's prescription for caregiving and hope can be found in surprising places and encounters.

When the Dubuque police chief announced his upcoming retirement, an article was written about him in the local newspaper. He shared one of his most memorable moments from his thirty-year career in law enforcement:

It was the face of a sixteen-year-old girl who died at the scene of a car crash. Chief Kim Wadding said, "I looked at her, and she was just so scared." It was obvious to Officer Wadding that the paramedics had tried everything to save her, but they couldn't. So Wadding decided to give this girl as much peace as he could for as long as he could. He locked eyes with her and said, "Just look at me. We're going to get through this. This is going to be OK. Just look at me." He held her, and they looked at each other as he watched her fade away. "It's a face you never forget," Wadding said. "And that's what keeps you going—those few seconds of comfort. I felt that she felt it."[33]

Many years ago, a friend introduced me to the writing of David Steindl-Rast, a Benedictine monk who also studies Zen Buddhism. Steindl-Rast, like many theologians, had searched his heart and mind and experience in a quest to define God. He ultimately defined God as "surprise," saying no other definitions can ultimately be sustained.[34] Because this story about Chief Wadding's memorable moment was so surprising, I looked prayerfully and deeply into this story, looking for God. What I found beneath the chief's words was Vaclav Havel's definition of hope: "Hope is not about believing that you can change things. Hope is believing that what you do makes a difference."[35] Chief Wadding could not change the fact that the girl would die, but he could—and he did—make a difference in that girl's life. And, clearly, that girl made a difference in his.

At a Healing Moments workshop for Alzheimer's caregivers, I shared Chief Wadding's story. A staff member from the Alzheimer's Association exclaimed, "She died! How is this hopeful?"

That's right she died.

Like this girl's injuries, Alzheimer's is terminal. Unlike this girl, however, who had only moments left to live, people with Alzheimer's can live with the disease for decades. Our challenge is to help those afflicted with Alzheimer's to get through the time they have—moment by moment.

As we help them, what then happens for us? As we live into the answer, we might find another surprise.

When I visited Iowa the summer after my sibling moved away, my intention was to assess the possibility of moving to Dubuque from Boston to be with Mom. Well-meaning friends and colleagues challenged the basis of my mission. They expressed disbelief and concern that I would consider leaving my established life and career opportunities in Boston and move halfway across the country to care for someone who barely spoke and, most of the time, didn't even know who I was. My initial response to this argument was, "Well, I still know who she is. And who she is needs me, now more than ever before."

As I spent more time with Mom and her neighbors in the nursing home, however, I began to question the premise that people with Alzheimer's don't know their loved ones. I saw the nursing home residents light up like fireflies when their sons, daughters, spouses, friends, and cherished caregivers came for visits. Faces that were often blank burst into smiles as soon as they noticed their loved ones approaching.

Etty was Mom's neighbor on the Alzheimer's wing of the nursing home. Her husband was away for the winter, and although they had spoken on the phone, she hadn't seen him for six months. On the first day he returned, he respectfully greeted her, asking if he could hug her. Etty cautiously hesitated but then agreed. He took her out for lunch, and when they returned, he kissed her good-bye and left her at the nurses' station. With a dreamy gleam in her eye like a teenager in love, she shouted out to everyone, "I'm going to marry that man!" She didn't remember that he was already her husband, but something in her knew they belonged together.

Perhaps her spirit recognized his spirit. That's what I felt was happening between Mom and me during our time together that summer. One afternoon, she was absorbed in looking at and touching the new clothes I had laid out on her bed earlier in the day. When I walked into her room, she looked up from the clothes. Quickly, she recognized me. I knew this from the wide smile that spread across her face. As she clutched her new flowered blouse to her heart, Mom's shining blue eyes looked at me— really looked at me. Then she said slowly but distinctly, "You. You. It's you!" Her face and eyes expressed awe. Hearing this, seeing this, I felt as if I was, at that moment, a visiting deity—or at least the most important person in my mother's world. It was a moment of pure recognition and belonging, even if she wasn't exactly clear about the relationship between us.

After those seven weeks with Mom, I returned to Boston in turmoil. My life in Boston was fulfilling and happy and I couldn't imagine myself thriving in a small town in Iowa. I sought counsel from respected friends, colleagues, and counselors, who mostly discouraged the move. Only my spiritual director recognized the longing of my soul to be with Mom, and she encouraged me to follow this call. The turmoil intensified.

One hot September day on a sunny beach north of Boston, I crouched at the shoreline and watched tiny sand crabs skittering in and out of the water. As my mind focused on the crabs, a calmness came over me and a question posed to me long ago during a session of the Life/Work Directions program[36] rose into my consciousness: "What would you do with your life if you found out that you had only six months to live?" A clear answer came quickly. I would finish my semester of school, keeping the commitments I had for teaching classes and workshops, and then I would go to Iowa. Then I asked myself another question: "If you knew that your mother would die in six months, what would you do?" Instant clarity: I would move to Iowa tomorrow.

Without doubt or delay, I began making arrangements to move to Dubuque. I completed my teaching and workshop commitments in Boston, spent six weeks during December and January in Iowa with Mom, and officially relocated in February. When friends and colleagues asked me why I was doing this, I explained that, when I arrived in Iowa in July, my mother couldn't get up from a chair without assistance. She couldn't walk, feed herself, or catch a ball. When I left in September, she could do all of those things and more.

I told a friend how I "cued" Mom to get out of a chair without assistance by telling her the steps in the process: "Put your hands on the arms of the chair. Now push up with your arms. Now push up with your legs."

He remarked, "Oh, so she has to relearn how to do things."

"That's not exactly it," I replied. "Mom's not relearning. Although she has the physical strength and ability to stand up, she doesn't remember how to initiate this action. I'm noticing her remaining abilities and then helping her to use them."

The sad truth was that Mom would not regain the capacity to stand up from a chair on her own. For a while, however, she could do this with minimal cueing, such as slight pressure on her elbow and the verbal suggestion, "Let's stand up now."

Persons with Alzheimer's have remaining abilities that are unrecognized, unused, and too often lost forever from inertia and atrophy. Mom needed me there to help her maintain her abilities for as long as possible. Sadly, it's often more practical and efficient for nursing home staff to lift a person from a chair than it is for them to offer cues, wait for the cue to register in a decaying brain, and then patiently allow the person to actually follow the cue and perform what has been asked. This quicker fix is detrimental to persons with Alzheimer's, because for them the old adage is especially true: If you don't use it, you lose it.

As my plans evolved to be with Mom during the home stretch of her life, I explained to inquiring colleagues and friends that, during the weeks I spent with her, I was making a significant difference to her well-being and quality of life. This mattered to me. I couldn't stop the course of Alzheimer's disease or change the fact that my mother would die, but I saw that, in the midst of these harsh realities of life, healing was possible—healing was happening. I felt that I was living Vaclav Havel's definition of hope; I believed that my presence in Mom's life was making a difference in important and meaningful ways.

As we search to understand what hope might mean for individuals and societies caring for persons with Alzheimer's disease, we need to consider various contexts for hoping.

One hundred years after Dr. Alzheimer discovered the mysterious plaques and tangles in Auguste D.'s brain, we are still hoping that science and medicine will identify ways to prevent, treat, and cure this disease. Advances in research into other diseases over time give us reason to expect similar strides in Alzheimer's research. For example, current science suggests that, although research has not discovered a cure, prevention might be accomplished by identifying "healthy brain" behaviors similar to the recommendations for preventing heart disease. These behaviors include attention to diet, exercise, stress-reduction, and proper sleep.[37] This kind of hope, based on logic and reason, offers some consolation to a fearful population.

Finding hope becomes more challenging within the context of caring for the millions of Americans who currently have Alzheimer's and the millions more who will have it by 2050. This reality is daunting and becomes even more so as we consider the impact Alzheimer's disease and related dementias have on tens of millions of family caregivers. These "informal" caregivers, who contribute millions of unpaid hours of care, often suffer significant financial loss and are susceptible to illness, depressions, anxiety, and often, early death.[38]

In the medical world, efficacy—a capacity for producing the desired result or effect—gives medical professionals and patients alike realistic hope that there are ways to alter or halt the progression of an illness. The concept of efficacy gives people seeking cure through medicine a belief that things will turn out well. Alzheimer's disease, however, has awakened us to the reality that hope is not synonymous with optimism, particularly if we are looking for hope in the usual places—such as the doctor's office—where this disease is a big question mark for everyone.[39]

In an effort to find someone or something that will change unbearable realities, most of us tend to look outwardly for hope. True hope for Alzheimer's, however, requires us to first accept the reality that humankind cannot bear: Alzheimer's is an unpreventable, incurable, degenerative brain disease. This reality invites us to consider suffering as a natural part of the human condition. On this topic, saints and poets, both ancient and modern, have insights to share. Julian of Norwich, a fourteenth-century Christian mystic, shares her perspective: "During our lifetime here we have in us a marvelous mixture of both well-being and woe."[40] Four hundred years later, poet William Blake expressed a similar life view:

> Man was made for joy and woe.
> And when this we rightly know,
> Through the world we safely go.[41]

From the springboard of these truths, hope inspires us to accept that life includes loss, decline, suffering, and death. This inevitability of the human condition becomes significant, personally and socially, in ways that have ethical consequences. Only by accepting the suffering of Alzheimer's, which brings us face to face with what theologian Teilhard de Chardin calls "a universal power of diminishment and extinction,"[42] do we have the option to overcome it and transform it into an experience that is, in essence, life-giving.

In the face of this universal power of diminishment, we realize that hope is not "out there." Hope is within every one of us. Through the practice of conscious and compassionate caregiving, we can alleviate the suffering of persons with Alzheimer's, and we can make a difference.

Caregivers often engage in power struggles with persons with Alzheimer's over life-changing, life-saving issues such as driving, attending adult day centers, bringing help into the home, and moving to care facilities. These complex struggles are often resolved only when something significant happens. For Mom, it was a car accident that took away her license and finally the pronouncement by the doctor that she was not competent to drive.

There is no one right formula for ensuring that these dis-

cussions go smoothly. Whenever possible, however, and pref-
erably before a tragedy happens, caregivers are encouraged to
enlist the support of someone the person with Alzheimer's considers to be in a position of authority: a doctor, lawyer, family
matriarch or patriarch, boss, priest, minister, or someone else in
a leadership role. It will be especially beneficial if these authority figures have sensitivity to and awareness about the dynamics
of Alzheimer's.

My friend Diane is a parish priest in a neighboring town. A
member of her parish, Miriam, was diagnosed with Alzheimer's.
When the time came for Miriam to move into a nursing facility, her daughter Jessica, an overburdened, single working mom
with three teenaged sons, couldn't cope with Miriam's resistance, and she sought Rev. Diane's help.

Before the move, Miriam's aging, sick dog had to be put to
sleep, and her messy apartment had to be packed up and cleaned.
The even bigger challenge was the need to convince Miriam
that the move was necessary, good, and above all, happening.
Jessica told Miriam that she had to move, but Miriam was not
having it. Because of the role reversal of authority, it was hard
for Jessica to convince her mother to take her seriously. When
the priest (a clear authority figure for Miriam) arrived on the
scene, however, and told Miriam that the move was happening, she accepted it, although she was devastated. Rev. Diane
witnessed Miriam's sadness by sitting with her as she cried and
comforting her with undivided presence.

Miriam didn't want change because she didn't realize that
things could be better. As Rev. Diane explained what would
be happening and how, Miriam became curious about many
things, including why she couldn't ask Jessica any of her questions without emotions exploding. Rev. Diane replied, "Because
this change is as hard for Jessica as it is for you." Indeed, moving persons with Alzheimer's and dementia to nursing homes
against their will is very hard for their families.

For over a week, Rev. Diane spent many hours each day with Miriam, explaining (and re-explaining) with kindness and compassion what was about to happen to her beloved dog, and the reasons for and details about the upcoming move. Miriam didn't want to leave her apartment, and she kept forgetting why she had to go. Rev. Diane calmly repeated the simple truth, "Because you have Alzheimer's, and you forget things sometimes. You need to be around people who can help you remember." Rev. Diane's calm presence each day kept the process moving forward—in baby steps—which helped Miriam get used to the idea of change.

One day, Rev. Diane engaged Miriam in a practical task. She arrived with an empty moving box for Miriam to fill with pictures to take to her new home. As they removed pictures from the walls, Miriam told stories of her life as she decided whether to take or leave each item. Rev. Diane helped Miriam identify the most important things to pack with a clear request: "Let's talk about things you'd like to take." Surprisingly, each list ended with "the coffeepot." Pictures and clothes and shoes and the coffeepot. The cat and the TV and the cactus and the coffee-pot. When Rev. Diane mentioned to Miriam that she noticed the coffeepot was on every list, Miriam exclaimed emphatically, "I love my coffeepot!" They had a good laugh together over having a meaningful relationship with the coffeepot. Humor, compassion, and simple truth were some of the ways that Rev. Diane made a difference for Miriam.

After one of her afternoons with Miriam, Diane shared with me how excruciating it was to witness Miriam's torment and to feel so helpless. This is the plight of most Alzheimer's caregivers. Diane, however, was soothed by hope when she received the gift of knowing that her investment of time and her kindness toward Miriam had made a difference. On the Sunday morn-ing when Jessica was moving Miriam to the nursing home, she brought her mother to church before they left town. As Rev.

Diane was greeting the parishioners after the Mass, Miriam came up to her, stopped, and looked right into Rev. Diane's eyes. Finally Miriam said, "It's going to be OK," tacking on the question, "Isn't it?" Rev. Diane took her hands and replied with certainty, "Yes. It's going to be OK." They shared a long, warm hug. Then Miriam smiled at Rev. Diane and walked out of the church into the beginning of her new, OK life.

As Alzheimer's disease progressed for Hob Hoblitzelle, he informed his family and close friends that he was thinking, "Maybe it's time for me to get off the bus." Although Hob received support if he chose to get off, he also received encouragement to seek out further guidance, once again from his close friend and wise Buddhist teacher Jim. The turning point came when Jim inquired about Hob's quality of life: "How much pleasure and meaning do you derive from life and give to others? . . . It seems to all of us that you are getting a lot of pleasure from life and giving a lot as well. In fact, I think you give a lot more than you're aware of. . . . You don't see or appreciate how deeply and lightly, with humor, you touch people." Pondering Jim's response, Hob's wife Olivia wondered, "How do any of us know, even remotely, when or how we touch the lives of others?"[43]

Knowing my mom's life story, I realized that she had not been protected, nurtured, loved for who she was, or encouraged to be all she could be. How then could she have passed this kind of love and nurturing on to me when I was a child? My spiritual intention in moving to Iowa to be with Mom was to love her in this lifetime so her soul would learn and remember love and be able to love in her future life. Through this intention, which I thought was all about me caring for Mom, I made the most glorious discovery. Naively, or arrogantly perhaps, I was convinced that I would be healing Mom's soul. Over time, however, I most humbly discovered that she was also healing me. Mom was making a difference for me. *She* was being hope—for me.

From the beginning of Mom's journey through Alzheimer's, she inspired me, surprised me, healed me, and opened my heart and my mind. She beckoned to me from across the threshold of Alzheimer's and invited me into her world in Iowa, where I built a wonderful new life for myself. Most importantly, Mom offered me countless opportunities to be present in the moment, to practice giving and receiving unconditional love, and to recognize the presence of God in every beautiful and terrible corner of life.

Caregivers as well as persons with Alzheimer's have opportunities every day to *be hope* for each other. It happens in between us—with a smile, a touch, and a loving look in each other's eyes. It happens through witness and empathy, responsibility and solidarity, and recognition and belonging. We can't yet change the prevalence or the course of Alzheimer's disease, but every one of us—caregivers and care-receivers alike—can make a difference in someone's life. We can *be* hope.

The Value and Beauty
of Every Person

While I was holding Mom's hand, sitting with her at Rhythm Time, the Friday morning activity at her nursing home, our eyes met and she smiled. We shook maracas and sang along to old familiar songs such as "How Much Is That Doggie in the Window?" and "Take Me Out to the Ball Game." My eyes, drawn away from Mom for a moment, gazed across the expansive room and noticed what seemed to be a sea of wheelchairs occupied by nursing home residents. The scene tugged at my heart. It looked like a sea of orphans. Most of the wheelchair occupants were diagnosed with Alzheimer's or dementia. The administrator of the nursing home had told me that 70 percent of their residents had some degree of dementia. For many nursing homes, this would be a low percentage.

While I was shaking maracas and observing the residents participate in this activity, my mind wandered, and I wondered why more family members weren't there, enjoying this experience with their loved ones. Being with Mom and doing this activity together was actually a lot of fun for me, and Mom clearly loved and appreciated my company. I saw this in her eyes and smile as I helped her participate more fully than she could on her own.

My wandering thoughts led me to recall a recent article in the newspaper. Advertising the annual Alzheimer's Association Memory Walk, a well-meaning, but clearly uninformed reporter used metaphors that I considered distasteful and offensive to describe this sea of persons with Alzheimer's disease. Through his narrow vision, the reporter saw "empty shells" and "octogenarian Beach Boys, able to mount the stage yet unable to present anything new."[44] Obviously, he had never been to Friday morning Rhythm Time! There was always something new happening among these beautiful old souls. On this day, Etty was dancing her version of what looked like the twist; Mary and Tom, a resident couple, were holding hands and looking at each other with moonie eyes as we all sang "For It Was Mary"; Susan was singing in German; Ruth offered to pay for everyone's lunch with the Monopoly money in her red purse; Mom and I were attempting a wheelchair polka; hands were clapping, feet were tapping, faces were bright with interest and joy.

Because misinformed media coverage could influence people to formulate opinions and stay away from family members and nursing home residents with Alzheimer's, I wrote a letter to the newspaper editor. I shared my perspective, letting the population of Dubuque know that, through my eyes, my mother and her neighbors were not empty shells. The newspaper printed my letter, and I was pleased to plant seeds for another perspective to bloom and grow.

The uninformed reporter, unfortunately, is not alone in his misperception. Writers of a network television program, *Grey's Anatomy*, allowed one of their characters, a doctor whose wife had Alzheimer's and lived in a care facility, to see and pronounce her as "gone." This was the writers' justification, I presumed, for the good doctor's affair. In reality, the one who was gone from the relationship was the husband.

A combination of misinformation and fear about Alzheimer's causes many in our culture to conclude that persons with

Alzheimer's are useless. From an economic perspective, therefore, they are seen as a burden for families and societies.[45] Many families and friends of persons with Alzheimer's are juggling priorities, and if a person is considered "gone," spending limited time and attention elsewhere becomes an easier choice. How I wish everyone could see what I see looking back at me from the sea of wheelchairs: beauty within vulnerability, in-the-moment happiness, gratitude for any kindness, earnest efforts to engage in life at every opportunity, and, especially for Mom and me, celebration for one more day together.

How I wish everyone could feel the warmth I feel when, at times, I experience the nursing home as being like a college dorm, where residents are friends on a shared journey to a similar destiny, looking out for each other and enjoying each other's company. After dinner one Saturday night, Mom and I were in her room watching *The Lawrence Welk Show*. Mom relaxed in her wheelchair while I stood behind her brushing her hair. Music, companionship, and peacefulness filled the room and may have drifted into the hallway. This, I think, is what sparked Etty's interest. Like a college girl from down the hall, Etty walked uninvited into Mom's room and smiled. She spoke words that didn't add up to a sentence, but I replied anyway with a warm welcome. She sat on Mom's bed. Etty and I exchanged a few more words; Mom looked at Etty with interest. Then Etty sprawled out on the bed, arms tucked up behind her head, feet crossed, making herself quite at home. I was delighted. I turned the TV so she could also see, and we all watched together for a while in the loveliness of silent presence. Soon Etty was humming along with the band.

Then an aide came in and tried to shoo Etty away, telling her this wasn't her room, telling me it wasn't sanitary for her to be lying on Mom's bed. I insisted that Etty could stay with us, right where she was on Mom's bed. We were having such an enjoyable visit. Before Alzheimer's, Mom was a very sociable person, and I was sure she shared my delight about her friend initiating this visit.

Empty shells? Unable to offer anything new? Not through my eyes. What I saw was pure gold, shining brightly.

The essays "Memory" and "Hope" in *God Never Forgets: Faith, Hope, and Alzheimer's Disease*,[46] were my first introduction to Stephen Sapp, professor and chairperson of the Department of Religious Studies at the University of Miami. These essays were so engaging that I was inspired to personally contact Sapp. He graciously agreed to a phone interview and shared the unique view of Alzheimer's disease he had gained over twenty-five years of study, combining ethics, theology, science, and personal experience.

During our conversation, Sapp surprised me when he started talking about how much he enjoyed eating sweet corn. I chuckled about this because he lives in Florida. What could he possibly know about corn? A person hasn't really tasted excellent corn until he or she has eaten an ear picked fresh from an Iowa field! As it turned out, Sapp wasn't really talking to me about corn. He was talking about whether and how our culture values elders and persons with disabilities, particularly those with Alzheimer's, whose potential is presumably used up.[47] Corn was his metaphor.

He told me how much he loved eating steamy, buttery sweet corn—on the cob, of course. After he's devoured the tasty kernels, he throws the cob away, believing as most of us do that it has served its purpose and is now useless.

With sadness, Sapp believes that most in our society assume that persons with Alzheimer's have no potential left, nothing more to give. Based on all the misconceptions about this disease and the observations we make with what ancient Hebrew prophets described as "eyes to see but do not see,"[48] it's understandable how we could mistakenly conclude that the potential of persons with Alzheimer's is all used up. As a society, we tend to devalue beings and things when their potential is not blatantly evident, and as a result, we could be tempted to discard, shut away, or ignore this population of people.

Then Sapp was back to talking about corn. The metaphor moved on to include revelation and discovery. This grain was first developed from teosinte, a wild grass, over seven thousand years ago by natives living in present-day Mexico. Since then, corn has accompanied people migrating throughout the world and has been cultivated into numerous varieties. Throughout the centuries, the potential for corn kernels (seeds) has multiplied exponentially, and thousands of uses have been discovered, including farm animal feed, pet food, antibiotics, baby food, condensed milk, sweetener for fruit juices, food starch, peanut butter, flour, alcohol, and even textile products.[49]

Until recently, when it was discovered that the cellulose biomass of corn stalks, husks, and cobs could be converted into ethanol fuel, these now valuable resources were seen as useless and discarded. It took humans almost seven thousand years of coexistence with corn to discover that stalks, husks, and cobs still have something to offer, even after they have completed their primary role of aiding in the production of corn kernels. More and more about the ever-increasing, ever-valuable potential of corn continues to be revealed.

As I considered this slow process of revelation and discovery, I realized that the inherent potential was there all along— waiting. Waiting to be discovered by the human mind. The corn didn't have the capacity to reveal its own value. In order to see the hidden potential, people actually had to look for it. People were looking for it. Most recently, we were desperately looking, particularly for alternate and renewable forms of fuel.

It's not the corn's fault that it has taken so long for more of its inherent value to be discovered. It's not exactly humanity's fault either. It took evolutionary time for science and technology to develop the capacity for recognizing and harvesting the fullness of the corn's potential. But most importantly, the realization had to dawn on the human mind that we need *all* of what corn has to offer. This kind of realization is often an inspiration for exploration and, ultimately, discovery.

So it is with seeing the value of individuals with Alzheimer's. Our whole world needs to recognize and respond to their still-hidden potential, and it's up to us—those who know and love them—to begin our own exploration, to discover value and meaning, and to reveal it.

As I continued to investigate Sapp's corn metaphor, it expanded even further to include cultivation. Although corn contributes monumental value to the world, it does not exist naturally in the wild. It can only survive if it's planted, cultivated, and protected by humans.[50] Similarly, as their abilities decline, persons with Alzheimer's can survive and contribute the value that has been divinely implanted within them, only *if* their lives are cultivated and protected. Cultivating their potential and protecting their hearts, bodies, minds, and souls is our divine purpose—as individuals and as a society.

Sue Bender, author of *Everyday Sacred*, offers another creative, if unlikely, metaphor. Bender's friend Gale Antokal teaches a graduate art class called The 100 Drawings Project. The assignment for this class is to take a single ordinary object and draw it one hundred times. After teaching this class for years, Antokal finally decided to join her students in the drawing project. She chose a white enamel kitchen pot as her object. In Bender's analysis, this intriguing project for art students requires them "to find new techniques, materials, and ways to work—to take risks and exceed limits."[51]

Bender observed Antokal as she worked on this project "for hours, day after day," seeing and drawing her pot, becoming familiar with it through constant studying, and ultimately becoming emotionally attached to it—even taking it on family vacations. My favorite artistic depiction was of the pot reflecting the "many tiny colored lights at night by the water's edge at Piazza San Marco." In the process of observing the pot as a model for artistic expression, Antokal had, without intention, imbued "this most ordinary object . . . with meaning."[52]

Bender reports that she "spent a lot of time daydreaming about Gale's pot." Ultimately, she concluded, "If there are one hundred ways to see an ordinary white pot, imagine all the possibilities for viewing with fresh eyes an 'average' child, an 'average' marriage. . . . If you can take a white enamel household pot and begin seeing it brand new each time, *you can do it with anything.*"[53] Or anyone! Just imagine the possibilities for viewing, with fresh eyes, persons with Alzheimer's.

At an Aging in America conference in Chicago, I was honored to meet Dr. James Ellor, a gerontologist from Baylor University and author of the essay "Celebrating the Human Spirit," in *God Never Forgets: Faith, Hope, and Alzheimer's Disease.* Confirming my observations and supporting my growing belief that people with Alzheimer's still have potential and purpose, Ellor writes, "I, for one, believe that the millions of [Alzheimer's] sufferers, who can no longer read, no longer speak, still have a thing or two they can teach us, particularly about the love of God."[54]

The idea that people with cognitive loss, who can't read or speak, have a thing or two to teach us sets up a contradiction for most of us. But contradictions are often the greatest teachers of all. For example, religious scholar John Dominic Crossan points out that in the Christian New Testament, the parables of Jesus consistently invite those *with ears to hear* "to experience the world differently, so differently in fact, that expectations about the way things normally go might be completely reversed."[55] Reversals in thinking have enormous potential to enlighten us in profound ways if we can become open to having our worldview shattered and to the challenge of reimaging how we then might live. Consider this possibility: Rather than being useless, people with Alzheimer's and dementia could be our most important teachers in the school of love and life. When our eyes are hopelessly resting on the obvious losses of Alzheimer's, however, this might seem impossible to even consider. But as we attempt to do so, keeping Bender's thought in mind could be encouraging: "Maybe the most sacred things are the hardest to see, because they are so obvious."[56]

Essential things are often obvious, *and* they are often difficult to see. Once recognized, however, they seem obvious. Consider the story of the Sufi dervish, Mullah Nasrudin:

> Every day for four years, Nasrudin smuggled valuable treasure across the border of his homeland, Persia, into Turkey. Because the guards saw him prospering, they knew Nasrudin was somehow hiding precious cargo, and they inspected every corner of his belongings, including the saddle of his donkey. They could find nothing. Many years later, after Nasrudin had moved away, he encountered one of the border guards, who asked him, "Please tell me now, what were you smuggling?" With a broad smile and proud laugh, Nasrudin replied, "Comrade, I was smuggling donkeys!"

The open secret about the value of persons with Alzheimer's is hidden to many, but for those determined to see, it will emerge into plain sight. Many of us are often so busy focusing on the endless details of everyday life that we miss seeing the treasure; therefore, when Alzheimer's caregiving is added to our everyday lives, it's important to slow down and simplify in order to focus. The kind of vision we need might be resurrected from lessons learned in childhood. Antoine de Saint-Exupéry's classic children's book *The Little Prince* offers simple, timeless guidance for recognizing the sacred in persons with Alzheimer's: "It is only with the Heart that one can see rightly; what is essential is invisible to the eye."[57]

When we look at someone who has Alzheimer's with ordinary eyes instead of our hearts, many of us may see someone whose purpose and potential are over, someone who would be better off dead, or someone who seems already dead. On national television, via his 700 Club, televangelist Pat Robertson claimed that Alzheimer's is "a kind of death."[58] Dr. Robert Stern, Boston University professor and Alzheimer's researcher, sees persons with Alzheimer's differently, and firmly refuted Robertson's comment: "A person with Alzheimer's is always alive, always filled with feelings, always able to connect at some level. To think or say otherwise is absurd, naïve, inhuman."[59]

If we look really closely at persons with Alzheimer's through the lens of our hearts, we see farther and more deeply than do the inquiring eyes of the scientist who studies the corn, the imaginative eyes of the artist who sees meaning in ordinary objects, or the grief-stricken, loving eyes of family members and friends. If we look through the eyes of one who is seeking connection with the creator and sustainer of life, we might be surprised by the potential and glory these individuals with Alzheimer's still possess. From the ancient world of fourth-century Rome, Augustine of Hippo, considered by many to be one of the greatest Christian thinkers of all time, tells humanity that "our whole business in this life is to restore to health the eye of the heart whereby God may be seen."[60] Shining out from within every person, including persons with cognitive decline, is the spark of divinity.

Through my unique perspective and experiences, I have noticed that persons with Alzheimer's have the potential to inspire us, teach us, love us, heal us, amuse us, befriend us, calm us, comfort us, touch us—physically, emotionally, intellectually, and spiritually—energize us, enlighten us, empower us, forgive us, nurture us, open our hearts, bring out the best in us, and bring meaning and purpose into our lives. We may be surprised to realize that persons with Alzheimer's still have the capacity to show us how to be humble, trusting, courageous, and receptive, to be authentically ourselves in this present moment, and to be guileless and innocent. We may be surprised to discover that, if we look beneath memory loss and declining cognitive and motor abilities, persons with Alzheimer's can reveal to us the true value of life—theirs and ours. Within their inherent and indestructible ability to give and receive love, their beauty and their value shine forth.

Caregiver Sol Rogers lives in Massachusetts. His beloved wife has Alzheimer's and lives in a nursing home. Out of a desire to help other Alzheimer's family caregivers, Rogers sent his story to the helpline office at the Massachusetts/New Hampshire chapter of the Alzheimer's Association, asking them to let others know his good news:

> I have a wife in a nursing home with an advanced stage of Alzheimer's. She can't get out of bed, can hardly move her arms, and can't talk at all. To get out of bed she has to have a large lift that requires 2 people to get her in a wheelchair. I visit her every day and had become very depressed, couldn't sleep very well, and my body was shaking. I thought I was getting a nervous breakdown and would end up in a hospital.
>
> Then an idea came to me (probably from God). I told the aide to have my wife in bed the following day when I came to visit. She got the OK from her bosses for me to get into bed with her. I took off my shoes, asked workers to get her as far over on the bed as they could so there would be room for me and got in. I cuddled close hugging her and kissing her and telling her how much I loved her. In the meantime I asked her if she loved me,

but no answer. Then I said to tell me yes or no. Then she said "yes," the first word she had spoken in a couple of months. I was ecstatic. I was never so happy in my life.

Now when I come to see her everyday, they have her in bed. I get in with her for about an hour. Then they get her up in a wheelchair. I am now a happy man. I am less depressed and sleep much better. I guess love does conquer all.

I would like to get this message out to the thousands of husbands and wives who would benefit from my experience. I hope you can help in this matter.[61]

In a conversation with Sol, he added a p.s. to his story: "After she said this 'yes,' Rita was talking again, and laughing at my jokes for about four months. Once I asked her if she thought I was handsome. She said, 'No. Cute.'" He laughed and hugged her!

As a spiritual director, I take seriously my intention to recognize and respond to the movement of the Spirit of Life in all aspects of creation. One evening, a particularly surprising and challenging experience brought to life for me Ellor's belief that persons with Alzheimer's can guide us into deeper relationships with God.

It was the holiday season. As I walked down the long corridor, admiring the festive holiday decorations, I noticed Renee. She appeared restless and agitated. As I passed by her chair on my way to the craft room, Renee leaned forward and reached out to me with her delicate hand.

Almost whispering, she said, "Can you come here? I have to ask you something."

Moving close to her and taking her outstretched hand in my own, I bent down and looked into her eyes. "OK," I said.

With grave sincerity, she asked, "Is Santa real?"

From the urgency of her expression and the firmness of her grip, I knew the answer to this question was deeply important to Renee, so I didn't respond immediately. I looked closely into her eyes, and there I saw the answer.

"Yes," I said, returning her firm grip. "Yes, Santa is real."

She relaxed her grip ever so slightly and replied, "I thought so. But they are trying to tell me there isn't one."

"Who's telling you this?" I asked.

"Well, I don't want to say," she replied. "I don't want to get anyone in trouble."

"Oh no. You mustn't tell then," I said, reinforcing her choice to protect the doubters.

Still clearly upset by the quandary, Renee leaned closer to me and asked, "But what should I do now?"

Time stopped. I took her hands in mine and looked deeply into her eyes. In that moment of true connection between us, I replied, "You just keep believing. You just keep believing."

"Yes," she said, taking a deep, slow breath. "Yes. I'll do that."

"Just keep believing," I repeated this over and over like a mantra, more to myself now than Renee.

"Thank you," Renee said, her sweet smile revealing a row of missing front teeth. "I feel so much better." She let go of my hand and sat back in her chair with a sigh of relief, peaceful at last.

Renee is not the real name of the one-hundred-year-old woman who asked me if Santa is real. I didn't know her name when we spoke. Although she also had Alzheimer's disease and lived in the nursing home on the same floor as Mom, I had never before met her or even seen her.

Receiving a question about Santa's existence from this stranger had caught me by surprise, and at first I wasn't sure how to respond. Mom was no longer talking, so my skills for verbally meeting persons with Alzheimer's in their world were a bit rusty. But I did remember the importance of being present in this moment and the healing implications of meeting persons with Alzheimer's in their current reality, which for Renee might have been Christmas, 1915. I did my best in a confusing and stressful moment for her, and she felt better.

After I left Renee and walked on toward the craft room to work on a project with Mom, I noticed that I felt better, too—light, peaceful, joyful—in the Christmas "spirit." As I reflected on my conversation with Renee, I realized it was both an endearing and profound experience for me. I felt inspired at a deep level. From the intensity of her question, she could have been asking me if there is a God. Given the course of Alzheimer's disease, every afflicted person—and their families and friends—might have spiritual doubts.

This encounter with Renee reminded me of David Steindl-Rast's definition of God, surprise. Everything about this conversation was a surprise for me: a one-hundred-year-old woman asking about Santa, finding the healing answer in her eyes, and the power of my own words to bring comfort to someone in confusion and distress. I was also surprised by my reply to Renee. It was an expression of my faith: In the face of doubt, fear, and resistance, keep on believing in the possibility of goodness.

After Mom went to bed that night, I looked for Renee to say good night but couldn't find her anywhere. For a fleeting moment, I wondered if Renee was real, if the profound experience had actually happened. Of course, she was real; of course it happened. A few months later, I officially met Renee and enjoyed her company for almost three more years. But on that night, my hope for Renee was that she slept peacefully, still believing that life can and does bring good gifts even in the midst of loss. I certainly slept well in this belief.[62]

When Mom began her journey through Alzheimer's, I was too terrified to even open a book about it. As her companion through the years, however, I have been given countless opportunities to confront my helplessness and fear. Somehow, I have managed to continuously welcome and embrace these opportunities. Within this embrace, I have come to see persons with Alzheimer's through the eyes of one who seeks meaning and value and beauty in every person and every experience of life. Subsequently, Mom and my new friends with Alzheimer's have guided me into closer relationships with them, with myself, and with God. I have seen their beauty and their value and have fallen hopefully in love with them. Through my love for them, I have discovered satisfaction in life beyond my imagination, beyond my hope.

I understand that to consider persons ravaged by a relentless disease such as Alzheimer's to be of value individually and socially, reversals in thinking and imagining are essential. In a culture such as ours, where youth and external beauty are practically worshipped, these reversals are especially challenging.

Every older and disabled person I've encountered has vehemently said, "I don't want to become a burden." Mom and her neighbors remind me that we may not have a choice about diminishing to the point of dependence, but what if caregiving for persons with Alzheimer's and dementia doesn't have to be a burden?

As I gazed out over the sea of wheelchair orphans at Rhythm Time, I thought of Victor Hugo's insightful words from *Les Misérables*: "The beautiful is as useful as the useful . . . Perhaps more useful." My attention returned to Mom and "The Beer Barrel Polka," performed with dedication by a woman who has played the accordion for more than fifty years. Mom's eyes followed me as I swayed and hopped in polka rhythm, careful to stay within her line of vision. She smiled and tried to tap her feet. I saw this tapping attempt, and my heart swelled with love and pride on her behalf. I smiled back. I remembered the prayer originally written by Augustine of Hippo: "Belatedly I loved thee. O Beauty so ancient and so new, belatedly I loved thee. For see, thou wast within and I was without."[63]

Redefining Self

When Auguste D. first met Dr. Alzheimer, she exhibited memory problems and described the anguish of her condition by saying, "I have lost myself."[64] Her medical records don't elaborate on what Auguste meant by her declaration, so to explore this, we can only speculate that the cognitive decline of this mysterious disease had brought its first identified victim to the point of wondering about life's most important existential questions: Who am I? What is my "self"? Who is my self? Where is my self?

Seventeenth-century French philosopher René Descartes's conclusion, "I think, therefore I am," expresses the common definition of *self* as it was understood by the traditions of Western philosophy and theology dominant in Germany during Auguste's lifetime.[65] Although this definition stills lingers in twenty-first-century American culture, Franciscan priest Richard Rohr asserts that Descartes' statement "was probably the lowest point of Western philosophy."[66] Neuroscientist Antonio Damasio evaluates the logic of Rohr's position and the lingering impact of Descartes's statement in his book *Descartes' Error: Emotion, Reason, and the Human Brain*. Through his important research, Damasio has brought attention to the valuable roles of the body and the emotions within the loop of brain activity and reason.[67]

In the context of societies where the self was, and still is, considered fundamentally rational, disembodied, and solitary,[68] it's understandable that Auguste D. and other persons with Alzheimer's experience memory loss and other cognitive problems as loss of self. I wonder, though, if an alternative understanding of self as relational were accepted as the norm and valued, would persons with Alzheimer's continue to experience their decline of cognitive memory and abilities as an existential loss of self?[69]

During the 1970s, feminist theologians and writers brought forth the relational understanding of self. Damasio explored a parallel definition in research first published in 1994. These alternate definitions of self, proposed by theologians and scientists, include our bodies, our feelings, our relationships, and our communities.[70] As we apply this more holistic definition of self to persons with Alzheimer's, we—and they—will discover that much of the self remains intact into the end stages of the disease. Within Mom, and within the hundreds of residents with Alzheimer's and dementia living with her at the nursing home, I met the self that remains throughout the long course of Alzheimer's.

The Embodied Self

As I considered the necessity of approaching Alzheimer's from the perspective of holistic healing, I became consciously aware that one of the body's remaining capacities was its ability to heal itself. On a quiet Saturday morning, from the deserted hallway of the nursing home, I heard a resident named Iris weakly calling for help. I peeked into the hallway from the door of Mom's room and saw Iris lying on the floor. I rushed to her side and saw that her shoe was untied. She must have tripped over her dangling shoelaces and fallen. Her face was already showing bruising, and she was crying in pain. After reassuring her that I would bring help, I sprinted to get the nurse. Because Iris couldn't articulate the source of a specific injury or her pain, a couple days passed before she was taken to the hospital and it was discovered that her arm had been broken in the fall.

Seeing Iris day after day, I witnessed her embodied memory for healing. The black-and-blue bruises on her face changed colors every day, to purple and red, then green and yellow, and finally they disappeared. At the same time, the broken bones in her arm, protected by a cast, were knitting themselves back together. In the exact amount of time it would have taken for my broken bone to heal itself—six weeks—Iris's broken arm was repaired. Her healing process was, for me, a shining demonstration that Iris and I were alike. In many ways, our bodies were similarly functioning and remembering. Throughout my daily observation of Iris's healing, what most intrigued me was the concurrence of healing and decay. Her teeth were continually falling out; she was losing weight and losing words; she was walking less. But by healing her wounds and various subsequent infections, Iris's body continued to reveal her aliveness.

Persons with Alzheimer's will react to physical pain throughout the course of the disease. One night while I was with Mom in Iowa during the moderate stage, she was washing dishes and something happened. I didn't know what, but she started saying over and over in a plaintive tone, "Little finger, little finger, little finger." She clutched her finger. I asked what happened, but she said only, "Little finger." I examined her finger; there was no blood. So I held her finger for a minute, applying pressure. Then, not knowing what else to do, I kissed it. This was a moment of confusion for us both. Mom couldn't tell me what had happened; I didn't know if her finger was broken or burned or pinched or bruised. I felt helpless and wanted to cry. Should I take her to the emergency room? While I was trying to decide, the pain must have subsided. Mom relaxed and returned to the dishes.

In the end stages of the disease, when Mom couldn't even say what hurt, she expressed her pain by grimacing, wincing, shaking, and when the pain seemed to be at its worst, her eyes rolled back into her head. At these times, she was unresponsive, her body limp. This was frightening to me, but Mom was taking care of herself. She knew exactly what to do to get through the pain, and she knew how to communicate her distress to those around her who had knowledge and observant eyes so she could get the help she needed.

In addition to reacting to painful sensations, persons with Alzheimer's respond appropriately to touch that is gentle and loving or brusque and rough. Various forms of gentle healing touch may have wide implications for improving the quality of life for persons with Alzheimer's. When Mom was in the hospice program, one of the benefits was a biweekly massage. The massage therapist told me that one of his male clients surprised his daughter by liking the massage. The daughter was shocked that her father allowed the massage therapist to touch him at all; that he liked it was beyond her comprehension. People with Alzheimer's who have previously resisted being touched might change their preferences, so it's important not to make assumptions.

Mom also appeared to love her massages, which were gentle, unlike the deep tissue massage many younger people use for releasing muscle tension. During her massages, Mom either kept her eyes wide open, watching every motion but resisting none, or closed them, wearing a blissful, peaceful expression on her face. Because she was in and out of the hospice program, she didn't receive massages regularly. In between professional massages, I continued offering her gentle, healing touch by massaging her face, neck, shoulders, hands, and feet.

Families and friends often wonder what to do when visiting persons with Alzheimer's, especially in the late stages as verbal communication wanes and other shared activities, such as playing cards or games, are no longer possible. During these stages, I chose to initiate an activity with Mom that I enjoyed, such as listening to music, watching a particular program on television, or just looking out her window at the beautiful countryside surrounding the nursing home. I would stand behind her and massage her gently. This became a shared activity that greatly enhanced our connection and brought us both comfort.

An opportunity for Mom to receive more healing touch came to me at the grocery store. Jenny was stocking shelves when I asked her a question about where to find a product. We started talking, and she mentioned that she was training to become a reflexology practitioner. For her internship requirement, she was looking for clients to practice on for free. Remembering that one of my spiritual direction teachers talked about her ministry of reflexology to nursing home residents, I volunteered Mom. Over the next several months, Mom received weekly reflexology treatments, which involved gentle massage of, and light pressure to, specific points on her hands and feet. After the first appointment, I arranged for the sessions to happen when I wasn't there, so Mom would have more company to make her days interesting. Jenny brought music and oil and her loving presence into Mom's life.

According to Dr. Robert Stern, "There is all kinds of research out there that the body and mind respond to touch in very positive ways. Whether it will actually have an impact on the progress of [Alzheimer's] is very unlikely, but providing someone with a connection…can only be positive for both."[71] I'm sure Mom enjoyed the healing touch of reflexology, and perhaps it helped to strengthen and heal her body in certain ways. She couldn't say how her body had been affected as a result of the treatment, but a special relationship had developed between Jenny and Mom. After Jenny completed her training program, she had to charge for her services, which we couldn't afford. Jenny continued to be a friendly presence in Mom's life, however. She sent cards. She visited and brought flowers. Mom smiled in her presence. Something had happened between them that had bonded them. Physical touch can reach beyond words, beyond reason, into the heart of who we really are and what truly nourishes us, relationship.

Damasio writes that our sensing body states are "inherently ordained to be painful or pleasurable." Without the reactivity of the body, "there would be no suffering or bliss, no longing or mercy, no tragedy or glory in the human condition."[72] It was my deliberate intention to assist Mom in experiencing bliss and mercy and glory for as long as she was living in her body.

The Emotional Self

Neuroscience researchers in Iowa have scientifically proven that emotional memory is retained by cognitively impaired persons whose brains have damage to the hippocampus, as is the case with Alzheimer's.[73] Having emotions and emotional memory shows without doubt that persons with Alzheimer's have not lost their selves. The research supporting this claim indicates that persons with cognitive loss can still experience an emotional stimulus in the moment. Although they cognitively forget the stimulus quickly, the emotional reaction generated by the stimulus, for better or for worse, will be retained for long periods of time.

Persons with Alzheimer's can experience and express a range of emotions throughout the course of the disease. According to Paul Raia, persons with Alzheimer's are very emotional and their emotions are usually appropriately expressed, given their interpretation of their experiences, although this appropriateness may not always be evident to or appreciated by observers.[74]

Sadness. One morning as I crossed the parking lot of the nursing home, I saw Etty's husband and their dog get into their car and drive away. When I got upstairs, Etty was standing in the middle of the hallway, weeping. She always recognized me as a familiar person, and when she saw me on this day, she walked toward me. I opened my arms, and she melted into my embrace. I held her as she cried. She seemed comforted, and when she stopped crying, she led me to her room to show me her stuffed dog. Nursing home staff, unaware of Etty's recent family visit and departure, wouldn't have been aware of the rational cause and effect of her tears.

Joy. Once a month, a country singer came to the nursing home and entertained the residents on Mom's floor. At the first concert we attended together, Mom's smile and the sparkle in her eye indicated obvious joy. To further demonstrate her appreciation and happiness, she attempted to clap. She raised her hands, moved her arms (by herself, without any cueing from me), and then clapped her hands together—once. She couldn't seem to remember how to unclap. And so her hands remained clapped as she continued to enjoy the music. She tapped her toe as her whole face smiled, and her eyes gazed with admiration at the singer. After the concert, I helped her stand (hands still together), and before I could direct her toward her room, she walked away from me, making a beeline toward the singer. I followed her and told him about her clapping effort. He took her hands into his, looked into her eyes, and said, "Thank you so much." Her smile told me that this event and this contact with the singer had made her day.

Gratitude. Maxine asked a nursing home staff member who was stocking the bathrooms if she could please have another roll of toilet paper. "Sure," the aide said, and she went off to get an extra roll. Then Maxine asked for another roll. This would make three in her bathroom, but the aide said, "Sure." After receiving the third roll, she asked if it would be possible to get a box of tissues. "Sure," the aide said again. When the aide placed the box of tissues in Maxine's hands, she smiled brightly and said, "Thank you so much. I think this is the nicest thing anyone has ever done for me." "How easy it was," the aide told me, "to make her so happy." Because many people with Alzheimer's can no longer verbally express their appreciation, this was also a particularly special, day-making moment for the aide.

Anger. In the dining room, most residents were accustomed to sitting in regular places. Maxine regularly sat at a table with a male resident and his wife, who was there to assist him with meals. One day there was an empty chair at their table, and I started to take it away so I could sit by Mom. Maxine erupted into anger: "You can't take that. That's my sister's chair. She's coming today." I had violated an unspoken dining room rule: Don't agitate Maxine. Don't try to help her eat; don't touch the chairs; and don't sit at her table! Not wanting to agitate her but needing the chair, I asked, "Well, do you think it would be OK for me to borrow this chair until your sister arrives? I want to sit by my Mom." "Of course," Maxine replied, showing a big smile sorely in need of dental intervention. "Thank you," I said. "Let me know when your sister gets here, and I'll return the chair." "OK," Maxine replied. Then she added, "Do enjoy your lunch with your mother, dear." Anger transformed into cooperation. Maxine was able to respond in a rational way to a clear request that made sense to her.

Fear. When feeling threatened or afraid, persons with Alzheimer's will express fear, and if they can, they will protect themselves. Marta, a high-school friend whose eighty-seven-year-old mother Gwen had Alzheimer's and was in a nursing home in Oregon, described an incident she witnessed. While trying to give Gwen her medication, the nursing home aide startled her. Because the room was crowded, the aide shoved a spoonful of applesauce and ground pills at Gwen's mouth from behind. Marta reported seeing in Gwen's eyes that she was startled and frightened by the sudden appearance of the spoon. With an instantaneous self-protective reaction, Gwen swatted at the air, hitting the aide's arm.

This aide didn't follow the prescribed protocol of getting Gwen's attention, making eye contact and explaining that she had a spoonful of applesauce and medicine for her. Perhaps this aide was unaware that persons with Alzheimer's often have compromised peripheral vision and that they eventually forget what spoons are and what they're for. What Gwen most likely saw and felt, therefore, was a foreign object being shoved into her face from out of nowhere. She was frightened and logically reacted by trying to protect herself.

Damasio's research confirms that human feelings "are not a luxury," and certainly not useless: "They serve as internal guides, and they help us communicate to others signals that can also guide them."[75] Gwen's immediate response was guided by the "emotional action program we call fear." This program, which was not taken away by Alzheimer's, "can get most human beings out of danger, in short order, with little or no help from reason."[76]

The Cognitive Self

When persons with Alzheimer's can no longer speak, we could easily conclude that they no longer can hear or understand what's being said to them and around them. On the contrary, long after persons with Alzheimer's have lost the ability to speak, they retain receptive speech: the ability to hear, comprehend, and respond to verbal language. Although many presume that persons with Alzheimer's are "absent of will," researchers refute this presumption by revealing that they, "surprisingly, still communicate through gestures and some spoken language in the face of 'quite severe deterioration.'"[77] Michelle Bourgeois, professor of speech pathology at Ohio State University, explains, "Persons with Alzheimer's will attempt to get us to understand with whatever remaining skills they have, so we need to stay with them, even when they challenge our limits of creativity, imagination, and patience."[78]

One rainy day at the nursing home, Mom and I walked together up and down the long hallways. The day-shift nurse was sitting at the desk as we passed by, and we stopped to chat with her. Being curious about people, I asked how long she had been working there. It had been over twenty years. She said that, when people learned she had worked in a nursing home for so long, they often asked her how she could work with the elderly. "Wasn't it depressing?" Mom must have heard "the elderly . . . depressing" because she clearly took something personally and was offended. She clenched her teeth, presented an angry look, and pounded her fist on the counter. The nurse and I looked at each other, stunned. The nurse took gentle hold of Mom's clenched fist and reassured her that she loved taking care of her. Then the nurse said to me, "Well, this has been an important lesson. I'll be more careful about what I say."

One night I arrived at the nursing home after dinner. The dining room aide had moved several chairs out into the hallway to clean the floor. Six women, including Mom, and one baby doll were seated in these chairs in a line against the wall. I asked the aide if I could play ball with them, and she found a multicolored beach ball for us. During the game with these six women—Etty, Lena, Iris, Ilene, Regina, and my mom—I learned something important about the capacity of persons with Alzheimer's to understand and respond. I started by throwing the ball to Etty. She caught it and threw it back. I threw the ball to Lena, the woman sitting next to Etty, and then all the way down the line. After each woman caught the ball and threw or batted it back to me (at this point Mom could only catch; she had forgotten how to throw), I started again with Etty. This predictability got boring for me quickly, so I decided to mix it up. I threw the ball to each woman in random order, not just once but a random number of times. I wanted to see if they were paying attention to the game. They weren't always, and often missed the catch or seemed startled when the ball hit their hands. Then I began calling each woman's name before I threw the ball to her, still in random order. As each woman heard her name, she immediately turned her attention to me. We made eye contact before I tossed the ball, and the catch success factor was almost 100 percent. So then I tried another experiment. Before throwing the ball, I called out "Mom," and not one of them, including my own mother, looked at me. This reminded me of one of Dale Carnegie's principles: "Remember that a person's name is, to that person, the sweetest and most important sound in any language."[79] After that experience, I began using Mom's given name, Jeanne, when I talked with her. I wasn't sure if she knew she was my mother, but I was very sure she knew that she was Jeanne. I wanted her to be comfortable around me, and calling her Mom might have confused her about our relationship. I continued this practice until the last couple weeks of her life, when I started to call her Jeanne-Mom.

Persons with dementia can understand and respond to requests and do things further into the disease process than we might think.[80] I discovered, however, that bringing out their abilities requires patience. In fact, nursing home life is a practice in patience for both residents and their families.

Alzheimer's, especially, calls for patience. When the weather cooperated, Mom and I went for walks outside almost every day. Since she lived on the third floor, an elevator ride was required. I remember the first magical time we walked to the elevator and I said to Mom, "Push the button down." At the time, I didn't know how much language she understood or how much she could do. As we stood at the elevator door, I saw her looking at the buttons—for a long time, it seemed to me. Then I noticed her arm slowly rising, her finger slowly pointing and finally pressing the arrow facing down. It took time, I assumed, for her brain to register the instruction and then to pass that instruction on to her body; then it took more time for her body to respond. Based on delayed responses, we could easily assume that persons with Alzheimer's capacities are "gone," and push the elevator button ourselves. Mistaken assumptions and impatience could prevent caregivers from knowing that persons with Alzheimer's can still do things and still want to do things.

My efforts to recognize and bring forth Mom's remaining cognitive capacities enhanced our ability to continue relating and enabled us both to feel joy over her accomplishments. I could see joy in her eyes and her smile, and it warmed my heart every time. Once inside the elevator, Mom could also respond to my instruction to push the button with the number of the floor we wanted, "Push one," I'd say. And beaming with pride, Mom would push the lighted round *1* button. With tears in my eyes, I beamed right along with her.

The Relational Self

Alzheimer's does not take away the desire or the ability to form and appreciate relationships. Although Ilene and Alice lived on different wings in the nursing home, they met during lunch in the dining room for the residents with Alzheimer's. Through some communication of their own, they came to recognize each other as compatible companions. They walked hand in hand down the hallways after lunch, having a conversation in sentences unintelligible to others but seemingly satisfying to them. One day as I passed them and said, "Hello," Alice reached out to me. She took me by the arm and shared very clear words of wisdom. "You just take it as it comes, and you give thanks to God for another day." Alice and I became good friends.

Most residents in the nursing home continued to manifest the innate human desire to connect with others and to be useful and helpful. They were actively engaged in helping to clean the dining room after meals. Mom washed the tables; John wanted to sweep; Regina was always gathering up the dishes. Mom and her neighbor Etty enjoyed pushing others in their wheelchairs. Once when an aide and I were helping Mom to stand up from her wheelchair, Lena saw us from across the hall. She came right over and offered to help Mom. We carefully guided, assisted, and supervised Lena in helping Mom to stand, and Lena seemed happy and satisfied to be of help.

Fulfilling their desire to remain useful and productive helps to maintain the self-esteem of persons with Alzheimer's. Keeping them actively involved in tasks at which they can succeed (such as folding laundry, setting the table, assisting with cooking, dusting, filling bird feeders, and watering flowers) helps them to sustain a good quality of life for a longer time.

After Miriam moved to the nursing home, her life was more than OK. In fact, she is flourishing. She voluntarily took on the role of assistant caregiver. Her interactions with the other residents involve helping them get comfortable, helping them stand and walk, and introducing people to each other. Rev. Diane suspects that, in Miriam's mind, she is now the person she wanted to be when she retired, "the helper." "So often in our conversations," Rev. Diane said, "Miriam talked about going back to work at Walmart because she loved her job there as 'greeter.' She was convinced that her mind would work better if she could do this. Interesting. It seems that she was right!"

During her most lucid moments, Daisy, who was ninety-four and in the middle stages of Alzheimer's, demonstrated (often to the dismay of the staff) that Alzheimer's did not necessarily destroy a person's capacity to affect and influence people and situations. Daisy did not hesitate to express her opinions. She was a reliable food critic, almost daily expressing her thoughts about the quality of the food she was served. If Daisy said, "This is the worst chili I've ever tasted," I usually asked the kitchen to send Mom a grilled cheese sandwich and tomato soup, her favorite meal. Since Mom couldn't tell me whether or not she liked something, I watched closely for her reactions and listened to Daisy's reviews.

One spring, the nursing home administration decided to replace the air conditioning system. Unfortunately, the timing coincided with an unexpected and severe heat wave in the Midwest. It was over ninety degrees outside and extremely humid. The third floor of the nursing home was almost unbearable. One particularly steamy night, as everyone capable of expressing their discomfort was doing so (mainly staff and family members), Daisy took on the cause of helping her neighbors. In the dining room, she loudly stated the obvious: "It is too hot in here! Somebody get a fan." All the aides ignored her. She kept demanding a fan. Considering her request to be disruptive, one aide tried to shuffle her out of the room. "I'm not going anywhere," Daisy assertively resisted. "I'm staying right here until you get some fans to cool off these poor people!" Which they finally did.

The propensity of persons with Alzheimer's to hold, feed, and care for baby dolls demonstrates their remaining instinct for nurturing. At first glance, giving dolls to elderly people and others with cognitive decline might appear demeaning. But dolls, teddy bears, and other soft, cuddly creatures bring them comfort and company. The night I was playing ball with the group of six women and one baby doll, I witnessed the nurturing instinct in action. The doll was sitting on a chair next to Etty. A rogue toss of the ball bounced off the doll's head and knocked her onto the floor. Etty reacted to this injury to the doll with horror, glaring at me like I was a murderer. She picked up the doll and cradled her. She carried the baby doll to her room, put the doll into her own bed, covered her up, and sat with her until it was bedtime. A retired teacher, Etty didn't have children of her own. She was, however, the most protective of the dolls and the most visibly reactive if any seemed injured.

Both men and women were attracted to the dolls. John had been a single parent to his seven children after his wife died giving birth to their youngest son. John loved caring for the baby dolls. His gentleness with them was remarkable. All of the residents regularly held the dolls; some would hold them, coo at them, and rock them for hours. They enjoyed talking dolls, crying dolls, soft dolls, and especially the ones that resembled real babies. Often the residents were more interested in engaging with the dolls than they were in eating. At meals, some of the residents attempted to share their food with dolls and teddy bears. It was messy but very sweet.

The instinctual energies of the libido are also still alive in persons with Alzheimer's. This became especially evident at Mom's nursing home when Rick came to work as an aide on her floor. Tall, dark, handsome, and very kind, Rick became an instant favorite among the many female residents. With dazzled eyes and giggly, groupie-like smiles, they followed Rick up and down the hallways.

Remaining energies of the libido can propose challenges as well. One resident forgot he was a priest. He flirted with and attempted to touch the young female aides. In response to such situations, many nursing homes offer the option of same-gender aide care. This was helpful to the aides in Mom's nursing home, because some of the male residents were flirtatious, even flirting with me. Some flirted in ways that were charming, some in ways that were gross. I didn't react negatively to either approach because I saw the flirting as a glorious reminder of humanity shining through Alzheimer's. When I knew this was a factor, however, I didn't get close enough to these men to risk being touched or grabbed.

Sometimes the residents flirted with each other. At lunch one day, Mom and I sat at a table with Bert and Regina. Bert thought Regina was his wife, and he repeatedly touched her hand and asked her to go to his room. Regina was shocked and offended. Blushing, she firmly responded, "No! I'm married." Her response was clear, but she was overtly flustered. After this episode, the staff seated them at separate tables.

Care facility stories of residents with Alzheimer's meeting and forming romantic or special relationships with other residents are common—even if they are married to someone else. In the movie *Away from Her*, the wife with Alzheimer's explains to her husband her attraction and connection to another male resident. "He doesn't confuse me," she said. Here is another reminder that we can maintain and nurture relationships with persons with Alzheimer's if, throughout the disease process, we can remember to meet them in their worlds.

Daisy's ninety-five-year-old boyfriend took the bus from downtown every day to visit her. One day at lunch, she told me they were engaged. "How wonderful!" I exclaimed. "And when is the wedding?" I asked. "It was supposed to be in the spring," Daisy replied. "But I might have to postpone that if I haven't lost enough weight to get into my wedding dress." At ninety-four, Daisy still wanted to look good for her man!

The Spiritual Self

Dr. Allen Power has worked as a physician and advocate for persons with dementia for many years. Drawing on evidence from his own experience, he concludes, "Even people with advanced dementia can experience well-being and growth."[81] A big part of my inspiration for choosing to be with Mom during the last part of her journey through Alzheimer's was my belief that the instinct and the potential for growth are in every one of us—from birth until death.

When I consider the natural instincts of people, including people with cognitive decline, my first thought is of growing—growing physically, of course, but also emotionally, spiritually, and more deeply into our humanity. A wise teacher once said that our purpose for being born is to help each other get through it all to the other side of life. I came to Iowa to help Mom get to the other side. I thought doing so would be a sacrifice, one I readily accepted. I was quickly surprised and humbled, however, to discover that, from a spiritual perspective, there was more to it. By helping Mom, I received much more than I gave.

Teresa of Avila wrote about spiritual growth and self before Rene Descartes was even born. She was aware of the limitations of the human mind, and her definition of self is considerably more expansive than his. "It seems to me," she writes, "that the soul is a different thing from the faculties and that they are not all one and the same." She continues, "Each of us possesses a soul, but we do not prize our souls as creatures made in God's image and so we do not understand the great secrets which they contain."[82]

As Alzheimer's disease progresses, it claims memory and cognition. It claims speech and movement. It does not, however, claim the soul, which, according to theologians going back to antiquity, is endowed with an immortal yet created essence. Those who define *soul* as "relational potential" have recognized this essence "even in the persons most severely affected by dementia."[83] If only we could know the secrets in the souls of persons with Alzheimer's, what treasures we might discover!

Perhaps anticipating a forthcoming, Descartes-like conclusion about the self as defined by mental faculties, Teresa writes, "I have sometimes been terribly oppressed by this turmoil of thoughts and it is only just over four years ago that I came to understand by experience that *thought is not the same thing as understanding* . . . [which] is one of the faculties of the soul."[84] In direct contrast to Descartes, she says, "The important thing is not to think much, but to love much. Do then, whatever most stirs you to love."[85] Indeed. Sam Keen echoes her thoughts: "In the depths of our being, in body, mind, and spirit, we know we are created to love and be loved. Fulfilling this imperative, responding to this vocation, is the central meaning of our life."[86]

Teresa's words are equally applicable and meaningful for caregivers and persons with Alzheimer's. According to Australian researcher Stephan Millett, if Alzheimer's caregivers "are helped to understand the inner life of a person with dementia, to look at them from the inside out, so to speak, they will be more likely to act for the sake of the individual with dementia and exercise sympathetic care."[87] Empathic caregivers are more likely to love than think; and effective, loving caregiving has the potential to advance both well-being and growth for care receivers and caregivers.

Because inevitable and relentless physical decline reminds us that death is ever near, we don't naturally consider the aging bodies and beings among us as valuable. We usually don't open ourselves up to embrace what Olivia Hoblitzelle calls the "grace of diminishment,"[88] and we rarely consider aging or illness to be a universal power that will ultimately transform into life-giving factors. In the fifteenth century, Dutch humanist theologian and Catholic priest, Desiderius Erasmus wrote, "Bidden or Unbidden, God is present."[89] Similarily, whether or not we accept and embrace the life-giving possibilities co-existing within the diminishments of Alzheimer's, they are still present.

In persons with Alzheimer's, I have witnessed an enduring resilient capability, and an ever-growing openness to giving and receiving love. In body as well as spirit, persons with Alzheimer's who have lost cognitive abilities still know that they are created to give and receive love, and they instinctively seek to fulfill their vocation.

Hannah, one of Mom's neighbors at the nursing home, was ninety-two. In the winter, she became ill and stopped eating. Everyone thought she would die. Although she was weak and thin, she surprised us by surviving. She began to eat again— even feeding herself. She once again smiled, walked, talked, and engaged with others. One evening as I walked into the dining room to assist Mom with her dinner, Hannah saw me and smiled. She extended her delicate, now bony hand to me. Her hair had been styled in the beauty shop, and her fingernails were like sun-drenched hot-pink peonies. I smiled with pure joy seeing her in this remarkable condition. I took her hand and held it. Our eyes met. Neither of us spoke, but the intimacy of the connection between our hands and our eyes brought tears to Hannah's eyes and then to mine.

"You're beautiful," she whispered in her slight, gracious southern drawl. My joy and my smile widened. I hugged her. She hugged me back, holding me close in a long embrace. When I looked into her eyes again, she drawled in a stronger voice, "I love you."

The stresses of my day drained out of me, and I felt transformed by the power of this surprising interaction. I took a long, deep breath and replied, "I love you, Hannah," feeling it to the depth of my being.[90]

The words of the Sufi mystic Rumi beautifully express why my encounter with Hannah touched me so deeply:

> The most living moment comes when
> those who love each other meet each
>
> other's eyes and in what flows
> between them then.[91]

In our society, we debate over which part of a human is most valuable: body, heart, mind, or spirit. Which deserves the most respect? The most care? The most attention? As I ponder this, it seems absurd to even ask the question. Until death, the parts are inseparable. According to Stephan Millett's research, "people with dementia continue to perceive and feel and to create a life-world"[92] in spite of diminishing cognition. Their souls—the immortal, created essence, the reflection of God, the relational potential, the "self"—remain strong and shining throughout their lifespan. Until their last breaths, people with dementia *are*.

Since love and relationship, more than cognition, define who we are and enliven our beings, I offer this alternative, inclusive, everlasting definition of selfhood: *I long to give and receive love—therefore, I am.*

Into Our Hands

Communication attempts by persons with Alzheimer's can sometimes be confusing for caregivers, but sometimes persons with Alzheimer's have trouble understanding our words and actions as well. Perhaps we talk too fast. Perhaps we're not facing them and making eye contact as we talk. Perhaps we don't know that they can't differentiate between consonants and that "Let's get in the car" sounds like an invitation to get in the "star." Perhaps we move too quickly or approach them in ways that feel threatening. Perhaps our body language or tone of voice doesn't match our words. Cognitively impaired persons will notice such discrepancies, reminding us that they may be more aware of our feelings than we are. Although they may not be capable of processing the implications of our feelings, words, and behaviors, they will feel and react to them.[93]

In confusing interactions, persons with Alzheimer's could be like scared improvisers who, seeking safety, try to block the offer. For instance, when Gwen was startled by the aide shoving a spoonful of pills into her face and swatted at the aide, she was trying to block an action she perceived as threatening. Gwen's intact emotional action program, cuing her to respond appropriately to fear, unfortunately, got her into rather than out of danger. Her self-protective swat apparently frightened the aide

103

and the entire nursing staff. Subsequently, they took big steps to prevent this action from happening in the future.

Their success in this endeavor still haunts my dreams. According to Gwen's daughter, Marta, the aide reported Gwen's action to the charge nurse as "acting-out behavior." This category includes behaviors that are considered potentially dangerous to the person, other residents, or staff. Apparently the aide considered a swat on the arm by a frail, eighty-seven-year-old woman as potentially dangerous. What happened next was standard procedure. Gwen was referred for psychiatric evaluation on the recommendation of the nursing home. The psychiatrist was told that Gwen was "acting out" by hitting people and refusing her medication. Perhaps that was an overstatement or a misinterpretation of the actual event. Gwen was admitted to the psychiatric hospital and prescribed antipsychotic medication and a sedative. Because she couldn't report side effects, she was overmedicated, perhaps even wrongly medicated, given recent medical opinions about using psychotropic medications for persons with dementia. When Gwen returned to the nursing home, she was confined to a wheelchair. She slept most of the day slouched and slumped over the side of the chair. She was awake, agitated, and disoriented during the night. Trying to get up on her own, she repeatedly fell out of her bed or chair and had bruises and cuts on her legs. She slept through many of her meals. Because she was diabetic, missing meals altered her blood sugar in medically alarming ways. Additionally, she retained fluids, and her limbs became swollen. Although she was very groggy, Gwen was taken to every meal. In semi-lucid moments, she tried to eat and drink, and she ended up gulping her fluids. Previous to her hospitalization, Gwen hadn't needed any help with her meals, so no one was helping her now, or even watching her. Another family member told Marta that Gwen was choking on her food and spitting up her gulped fluids. Soon she aspirated both food and fluid, and developed aspiration pneumonia. Three weeks after the incident with the medication aide, Gwen was dead.

In this chain of events, Gwen was not the only scared improviser. The nursing home staff and administration and the doctor who medicated Gwen all responded to perceived aggression in ways that contributed to the tragic outcome.

"In reality," Keith Johnstone tells us, "everyone more or less chooses what kind of events will happen to them by their conscious patterns of blocking or yielding. [An improvisation student of Johnstone's] objected to this view by saying, 'But you don't choose your life. Sometimes you are at the mercy of people who push you around.' [Johnstone] said, 'Do you avoid such people?' 'Oh!' [the student] said, 'I see what you mean.'"[94] Persons with Alzheimer's, however, are at the mercy of the benevolent/evil, informed/ignorant world. They don't have the option to avoid caregivers who push them around. Nor do they have the ability to say what they need, object to mistreatment, or require or request that caregivers become educated about Alzheimer's disease so they can be communicated with clearly and cared for properly.

Marta shared the day-to-day details of Gwen's condition with me, and over those three tragic weeks, asked many times, "What would you do?" Unfortunately, my responses didn't have much impact. Marta's stepfather, who was in his late eighties and somewhat confused, was Gwen's "responsible party" at the nursing home. He was, therefore, the only one empowered to make medical decisions on her behalf. Like most family members of nursing home residents, he consistently approved the recommendations of the nursing home. Although Gwen had other children, Marta was her mother's most consistent companion. She encouraged her siblings to try to influence their stepfather, but they didn't want to upset him with challenges.

During Gwen's last weeks, Marta visited every day, becoming frantic because she was powerless to help her mother. She was angry about what had happened with the medication aide and distraught by the outcome of her mother's attempt at self-protection. Marta didn't want her mother medicated in the first place, but because she wasn't the official decision maker, she had no say about her mother's treatment. Because of the gulping, choking, and swallowing problems at meals, Marta moved mountains to finally convince her stepfather to attain a speech therapy evaluation for Gwen. This resulted in dietary changes to softer foods and thickened liquids, which, if implemented sooner, could have prevented the pneumonia that caused Gwen's death.

While keeping vigil at Gwen's deathbed, one of Marta's brothers admitted that he thought her dying was for the best. He then said that living with dementia was no kind of life. This attitude, shared by many in our society, is probably the reason why these sudden deaths of previously healthy individuals with dementia remain uninvestigated, and why care centers remain uneducated about the specific needs of this population.

Each family touched by Alzheimer's will have experiences of conflict or cooperation that are as unique as the manifestation of the disease process. Caregiving responsibilities often bring out family conflicts that have been dormant for years, and invariably will separate those who can and can't handle it.[95]

Conflict within my own family complicated my desire to care for and accompany Mom during her journey through Alzheimer's. My sibling and I had parted ways almost thirty years earlier over disparate recollections of my childhood experiences. However, I had been told that Alzheimer's sometimes has the ability to bring families together, so I was open to this possibility. Our vastly different ideas about Mom's needs and what constituted appropriate care for a person with Alzheimer's, unfortunately, widened the gap. My sibling, who was living with Mom during the onset of the disease, believed that preserving

Mom's sense of independence was the top priority. Preserving autonomy is an important approach in the early stage, but when the progression of the disease puts a cognitively impaired person in danger, appropriate interventions become essential.

During my weeks with Mom in 2004, when she was in the early stages of her disease, I perceived her to be in danger. We went for a walk one afternoon, and when we reached a busy intersection, I paused to look both ways for oncoming traffic. Mom, however, pulled me by the hand into the street, and without looking started to cross.

"Wait," I said. "There are cars coming."

"That's not a problem," Mom answered. "Cars have to stop for me."

I recognized other potential hazards to Mom's well-being. If her meals were not prepared for her and her eating was not monitored, she probably didn't eat anything all day except candy from the bowl kept on the dining room table. Allowing her to have unrestricted access to alcohol, to use the stove unsupervised, and to wash dishes without having someone to check the water temperature seemed fraught with opportunities for injury. When I heard stories about Mom walking the dog and getting lost during below-zero days of winter, I really worried.

I insisted on taking Mom to physicians for an evaluation so her condition and her needs could be better understood as we determined a course of care. Through later study, I learned from gerontologist and theologian James Ellor that "the first place for advocacy" for a person with Alzheimer's is "ensuring that the impaired person has proper diagnosis of the disease."[96] I felt validated and relieved that I had followed my instincts and was able to at least do this to care for and protect Mom.

From my first encounters with Mom after the onset of Alzheimer's, I felt able and willing to handle her care. However, my sibling had acquired medical and financial power of attorney for Mom, and I was, like Marta, cast into the role of powerless bystander. For several years I was unable to care for my mother in any meaningful way.

After my sibling moved, the path became clear for me to relocate to Iowa and become Mom's on-site companion and advocate. Although I was now living two blocks away from Mom, my sibling, who lived far away and visited rarely, didn't want to relinquish control over her care. It made logical sense to me that, as the person who was in the nursing home every day spending time with Mom and interacting with the staff, I should be the decision maker. After much soul searching, many sessions of legal counsel, great financial expense, and several court hearings, I was named Mom's legal guardian. Family conflict persisted, however. Although I grew weary of legal wranglings, I knew at a deep level that this struggle was part of caring for Mom. Knowing what had happened to Gwen and accompanying Marta through her frustration, despair, powerlessness, and loss, I knew that my legal expenses, the emotional turmoil, and the conflict with my sibling were unquestionably worthwhile.

My new role as guardian, however, brought me face-to-face with decision making that could prolong or shorten Mom's life. The awesomeness of this responsibility caught me by surprise. In several situations, I anguished over what to do. Mary Anne, another caregiver who had been through similar experiences and feelings, coached me by saying that, no matter what I decided, I would probably feel some despair and guilt. Hearing this was oddly comforting. I hoped that Mom's time for death would be inevitable and obvious regardless of what I decided. Thankfully, it was so.

A basic necessity of care for a person with Alzheimer's is a committed and involved companion tenderly giving love and attention, and an informed advocate fiercely monitoring medical, in-home, and nursing home care. Two years after the death of his mother May, my friend and colleague Steve spoke with a tinge of grief about his own "reserved, nonconfrontational" personality.

Steve has spent his life being an impassioned political advocate. Consequently, he was surprised and disappointed by his inability to fiercely advocate for his mother on a personal level. In one instance, assisted by his wife who is a nurse, Steve did successfully fight to prevent the nursing home and doctors from prescribing psychotropic medications to manage May's "behaviors." Steve was very clear on that his mother was not the behavioral problem; the aides caring for her were. He was able to protect his mother in the way Marta could not protect Gwen. Ultimately, however, he couldn't protect her completely. One of the aides "let it slip" to Steve that May was given too much of a particular drug and that her kidneys were compromised and failing as a result. This would eventually lead to her death. Feeling defeated, he surrendered the fight and chose to be completely, compassionately present at his dying mother's bedside. He still carries within his mind, however, the imprinted images of incompetence and neglect that harmed his mother, and wonders if he should have pursued legal action against the hospital and the nursing home. Within his heart, he carries regret for his lack of fierce intervention on his mother's behalf, believing that he could have made different, better decisions for her.

As the understanding of what constitutes quality care for persons with Alzheimer's improves, care facilities are also improving. Even though we may meet resistance from nursing home staff, family members and guardians must speak up on behalf of persons with Alzheimer's because they can't advocate for themselves. Although many of us do try to be proactive advocates, not much seems to change in the short term. Some brave family members report infractions to state agencies, but they are generally able to effect change in only the most egregious cases. The more timid family members complain to friends but never to the nursing home administrators for fear of retaliation by staff against their loved ones. I was shocked to consider this possibility of retaliation, but apparently it happens in spite of a Resident Bill of Rights in most facilities promising that complaints can be voiced without fear of negative consequences for residents.

There were known incidents of abuse in Iowa care facilities during the years when I was Mom's companion at the nursing home. One male aide had molested female residents with dementia all across the state. He was fired from several nursing homes and eventually caught and prosecuted. No one wants to think about these possibilities.

We take our loved ones with Alzheimer's to state-inspected care facilities, expecting them to be cared for and safe. Although this expectation is reasonable, it is not always satisfied in the ways we want or in the ways our loved ones need. Even if things don't seem to change after we voice concerns and complaints, this doesn't mean that family members should give up and become silent. Our loved ones with Alzheimer's need us to speak for them. A staff member from the Alzheimer's Association advised me to advocate assertively for Mom. She said I would know my advocacy on Mom's behalf was effective if, when Mom passed away, the nursing home administrators were happy to see me go. I'm quite sure they were!

Steve, Marta, and all caregivers who do our best need to be kindly reminded that we have shared our tender hearts with our loved ones. Both Steve and Marta were attentive, compassionate caregivers for their mothers. They felt their mothers' suffering and sought to relieve it. Their care "healed" their moms. Hopefully, this awareness will help—in time—to heal them as well.

My family's story of conflict, Steve's story of regret, and Marta's story of helplessness are not unique. Numerous family members of persons with Alzheimer's have shared similar haunting stories with me. Unfortunately, the neglect, abuse, and financial exploitation of persons with Alzheimer's is much more common than any of us would like to think.

The abuse and exploitation of New York socialite and philanthropist Brooke Astor by her son Anthony Marshall made headlines across the country. In 2009, the ABC news program *20/20* heightened my awareness about the exquisite vulnerability of persons with Alzheimer's. Philip Marshall, Brooke Astor's grandson, recognized the neglect and abuse that his grandmother was enduring under his father's care. Encouraged by Brooke's friends to "do something," Philip reluctantly filed a petition to challenge his father's control and to become his grandmother's guardian and conservator.[97]

Knowing that every family conflict of this nature begins and ends in heartache, Philip Marshall and I shared the same internal turmoil: We wanted to care for our loved ones with Alzheimer's, but we didn't want to drag delicate family issues into the court system and thus into the public view. At the beginning of the Marshall family conflict, Philip naively hoped it could all happen quietly. He had no idea the heartache at the end would include nationwide news coverage and his father being sent to prison for financial exploitation of a dependent adult.[98]

Because many caseworkers from the Department of Human Services still hold the attitude that elder abuse concerns are a family matter that can and should be resolved within the family,[99] most of these cases never reach a prosecutor's office. The millions of dollars involved in the Astor conservator petition, however, caught the attention of the New York City District Attorney's office, and I was exceedingly grateful for the media attention to this story. Philip's courage gave me strength to continue my efforts to retain the legal right to decide what was best for Mom.

As I tried to understand the process by which abuse could develop as Alzheimer's makes people vulnerable, I was once again enlightened by James Ellor:

> [For family members] whose relationship with the senior have been difficult or abusive there is a sense of unresolvable anger . . . the lack of resolution can turn into vengeance when the angry family member becomes legally responsible for the person with Alzheimer's. It may also turn into neglect, a result of the deep conflict of emotions between a feeling of filial responsibility and anger that enveloped the relationship.[100]

From the reports about the relationship between Anthony Marshall and his mother, abuse in childhood and unresolved anger certainly could have been at the root of his neglect, abuse, and exploitation of his mother.

Current accurate statistics regarding the prevalence of elder abuse in America are unavailable. The most recent national survey was conducted by the National Center on Elder Abuse in 2004. The NCEA defines a "vulnerable adult as a person who is either being mistreated or in danger of mistreatment and who, due to age and/or disability, is unable to protect himself or herself."[101] According to Stephen Post, persons with Alzheimer's are a particularly vulnerable population of elders "in need of special protections from those without dementia, who are capable of a myriad of abuses of power."[102] In a 1991 article about elder abuse, E. T. Lucas describes the still-chilling reality: "People with dementia . . . are socially outcast, unwanted, marginalized, and oppressed. A remarkable amount of elder abuse and neglect falls upon people with dementia, not just because caregivers are exhausted or ignorant, but because persons with dementia are defenseless and easily victimized."[103]

When Mom moved to the nursing home, a zippered change purse disguised as a small stuffed frog survived the garage sale of her life and moved with her to the nursing home. This frog's belly held a religious medal Mom had put there years before and some coins I put there for card-playing wagers and for treats from the ice-cream truck. One day, on our way to get ice cream, I opened the zipper of the frog purse (which had been kept on Mom's bookcase with other stuffed animals) and found that all of her money was gone. Presumably, one of the staff had realized the frog was a change purse and taken the money. This is a clear example of persons with dementia being defenseless and easily victimized. Even if Mom had seen someone taking her money, she couldn't have identified the thief.

Although people with Alzheimer's are victims of physical, emotional, sexual, and financial abuse, "harm" to this vulnerable population can also result from "the absence of love and care," according to Post.[104] Without question, taking pocket change from someone who can't speak represents the absence of care as well as the absence of respect and regard. If Mom was awake at the time of the theft and witnessed someone violating her in this way, it surely caused harm to her heart and her spirit. The experience may have left her feeling fearful. This type of theft happens so often in nursing homes that residents are warned to keep valuables in the safe. A police report in the local newspaper stated that after a nursing home resident had died, a diamond ring worth over $10,000 was removed from her finger before the family or the funeral home staff arrived. The perpetrators of these small and large violations are rarely identified.

It's notable that Mom's religious medal was left behind in the zippered belly of the frog. Since it was the same size as a coin, the theft must not have been hurried.

National research conducted by the Illinois Department on Aging suggests that "elder abuse is seriously underreported because most people aren't informed, don't want to get involved, or don't know how to report an abusive situation." The report describes some of the challenges involved with protecting vulnerable elders from abuse:

- Only one out of thirty cases of elder abuse is reported. A woman interviewed in the film *Silent Crisis* reported being robbed of her life savings by her trusted, very wealthy daughter. The elder woman initially resisted telling anyone because she was ashamed and didn't want people to know that her own child had done this to her.

- Thirty-eight percent of reported abuse cases concern elders who are living with their alleged abuser. This represents a difficult challenge for social service caseworkers for gathering information and developing and monitoring a care plan.[105]

I met Felicia at a dementia care conference in New England. Her father was living in the southeast with Felicia's brother. A local social worker at a senior center noticed some problems and filed a complaint of neglect with the Department of Human Services (DHS), and caseworkers initiated an investigation into her father's care. Throughout this investigation, relatives continually contacted Felicia with alarming reports about her father's care and condition. Felicia tried to intervene, but her brother told her to stay out of it. Although she didn't completely comply, Felicia kept her distance because she was afraid of her brother's volatile temper.

When Felicia heard her father had lost an alarming amount of weight, she ordered Meals on Wheels for him. After a few meals, her brother cancelled the service, explaining that their father didn't like the food and it was a waste. Felicia asked her father if he liked the food delivered by Meals on Wheels, and he said, "It's better than nothing." Indeed, it is. When Felicia heard that her father wasn't taking his Alzheimer's medication, she attempted to have visiting nurses come. They weren't allowed in the house. This was also the case for the needs assessment ordered by her father's physician.

After listening to the stories from her relatives, Felicia asked them to repeat to the DHS caseworkers what they had told her. Not one of them agreed to do this. Like a chorus in a song, each person responded to Felicia's request to talk to DHS with the same words: "I don't want to get involved." Their reasons varied. One elderly relative told Felicia that she was afraid there would be consequences to her for speaking to "authorities." Felicia understood and accepted their decisions, but receiving their well-meaning reports of her father's unmet needs only made things worse for her. Having more information increased her concern, and her inability to intervene in a meaningful way increased her feelings of helplessness and despair. Her father continued to suffer, since DHS took no action.

Hearing about Felicia's experience helped me to understand German theologian Dietrich Bonhoeffer's words about the need for resisting the Nazis: "Silence in the face of evil is itself evil. . . . Not to speak is to speak. Not to act is to act."[106] Like many vulnerable and marginalized populations, persons with Alzheimer's continue to suffer because of the silence and inaction of others.

Unfortunately, staff members in nursing homes who witness their colleagues mistreating or neglecting residents most often say nothing. One aide in a nursing home saw another aide hit a defenseless woman in the bath. By the time the grapevine informed the management about this incident several months later, the abusive aide had moved out of town and the woman had died. The aide who had kept quiet was immediately fired. He didn't speak up at the time, fearing retribution from the abusive aide. He learned, however, that there are consequences for not speaking up as well.

Steve and I, and others who advocated for our loved ones with Alzheimer's living in nursing homes were shocked by some nursing home and medical professionals' neglect, abuse, and objectification of this population.[107] Steve experienced it as "inhumanity." I experienced it as appalling and fought to make changes and healing choices, at least for my mother.

During Steve's investigation of nursing home placements for May, as well as the years he spent as his mother's companion and advocate, he became aware of classism in the world of Alzheimer's care. In some parts of the country, elders with financial resources are able to live in newer, cleaner, better-equipped facilities with private rooms and more highly trained, more caring staff. Many facilities in Massachusetts that accepted Medicaid residents tried to convince me that housing four residents with Alzheimer's in one room was good for them. "They tend to isolate, so we don't let them spend much time in their rooms. And when they are in their rooms, they aren't lonely." This was definitely a good financial plan for the for-profit nursing homes, but newer recommendations for caring for persons with dementia would not support their rationale.[108] In other parts of the country—Iowa, for example—some nonprofit facilities provide each resident with Alzheimer's a private room and bath. The administrators cite "dignity" as their rationale, and there is no differentiation due to Medicaid status.

In most areas of the country, elders without any financial resources or without any concerned family members will be taken care of—perhaps in lesser-quality facilities, perhaps in fabulous ones—by federal and state monies through Medicare and Medicaid. It is critical that we continue to support our vulnerable elders through these programs.

Contemplating the prevalence of and various explanations for elder abuse, particularly the issue of unresolvable anger, I recognized the deep significance that leaving home had for my own healing and, therefore, for Mom's healing. Some people, aware of the intense vulnerability that is characteristic of Alzheimer's, see persons who can be easily manipulated, abused, and exploited. Others want to protect these vulnerable people. Between these polar opposite responses is a vast range of intentions toward vulnerable populations, including complicated, sometimes unconscious, motivations for caring. Acknowledging and exploring our own confusing feelings can present opportunities for caregivers to experience meaningful personal growth and to expand our relationships with our loved ones.

When my life journey intersected with Mom's Alzheimer's diagnosis and I touched the true meaning of vulnerability, something surprising and completely unbidden occurred. Witnessing Mom transform from an empowered, competent, independent woman to a confused, vulnerable, dependent, diminishing elder caused my heart to instantly widen. My heart ached to protect her and to care for her.

Had the intersection with Alzheimer's happened during an earlier phase of my life's journey, however, my heart would not have guided me to Iowa, into painful family dynamics to care for Mom. After leaving my abusive childhood home thirty-three years earlier, I wandered in a wilderness of despair that involved denying my pain with substance abuse and other addictive behaviors. In my late twenties, overcome by unhappiness, I started therapy and made a deliberate effort to embrace my feelings and resolve my anger at my mother for not protecting me. It was a long, difficult, painful process.

I have a distinct memory of a conversation with my doctor about my relationship with Mom that happened about fifteen years before she was diagnosed with Alzheimer's. I was wondering about the wisdom of staying in contact with her, given that most of our conversations and visits resulted in long-lasting despair for me. My main question focused around Mom's assets, even though she was not a wealthy person. Would she still leave me something in her will if I broke off contact?

My doctor responded with practicality: "If your mother lives long enough, she will probably require some kind of nursing home care, and most likely all of her assets will be used for her long-term care needs. So don't let money be your guide in this. Stay connected with your mother *if* you want to, *if* doing so is helpful to your healing." At that juncture, I chose to maintain contact with Mom from a distance that felt safe to me. Although I was angry at her and hurt by her constant rejection of me, my desire to love her was not extinguished. And I never stopped wanting her to love me.

My doctor's practical prediction came true. By the time Mom died, all of her financial assets were gone.

After Mom visited me in Maine in 2003, I revised my own will to include a trust for her care, should she need financial support. My heart had opened to her and widened enough that I wanted to provide for her physical safety. Being in her presence, however, and caring for her myself—these options didn't enter my heart or my mind.

A year later, when I spent time alone with Mom in Iowa and intimately touched her world, I more fully witnessed and experienced her vulnerability. When she recognized my kindness and asked me to stay and take care of her, my willingness emerged and did not retreat. After another three years, I made sacrifices and overcame obstacles to move to Iowa and care for her.

My desire to do this amazed me, and even more, my willingness. Many who knew me and who knew the details about my childhood and my historically troubled relationship with my mother were stunned and disturbed by my decision. By acknowledging and resolving my anger, I became open to caring for Mom and thereby transcended the past, rooting myself in the compassion I felt for her in the present.[109] Many people in Iowa who witnessed my commitment to Mom's care remarked to me, "She must have been such a wonderful mother, that you would care for her so dearly." I smiled, leaving them with their own conclusion. I have learned that the reasons for caring, or not caring, for a family member with Alzheimer's are as unique as every family's history and every individual's healing journey.

I met Coleen at Mom's nursing home, and we became friends and companions on the journey through Alzheimer's. Her mother Ilene lived across the hall from Mom. We all shared many meals and joyful times. We also shared our challenges with life and Alzheimer's.

As Ilene began to show signs of "something wrong," she resisted Coleen's presence in her life. Ilene was angry and directed her anger at her daughter. She accused Coleen of causing the problems she was having and manipulated other family members into doubting and criticizing Coleen. In her fear and confusion over the changes she was experiencing, Ilene lashed out at the person closest to her, perhaps believing that pushing Coleen away would resolve her own difficulties. Although Coleen stepped back and asked her brothers and sisters-in-law to watch over her mom during this time, she was not pushed away. She was always there in the background—aware, waiting, and ready. One day Ilene's resistance was over. She called Coleen and asked her to come. Coleen left work and went immediately to her mother's side. Ilene said sadly, "I think something is wrong." Coleen replied, "I do too, Mom. I do too. But whatever it is, I'll be here. And we'll get through this." For over fourteen years as her mom's dependable companion and advocate, Coleen kept the "vow" she made to her mother that day.

"The truest test of any society," according to French philosopher Simone de Beauvoir, "is how it treats the aged, those who are an unwanted reminder of our frailty and mortality."[110] Alzheimer's disease, like nothing else we have yet experienced, has a profound way of shining a light on the truth of who we are—as individuals, as communities, and as a society. Alzheimer's can bring out both the best and the worst of human nature.

My friend and ministerial colleague Carl Scovel pointed out that one important reason a society cares for its vulnerable people is that we all witness this and can then trust that we too will be cared for when we are in need.[111] There comes a developmental point in Alzheimer's when those afflicted will have no choice but to completely trust others, us, for their support and care.

Clinical social worker Marty Richards explains that they trust us not out of desire and not because we have earned their trust but because of the pure necessity to do so.[112] At every moment, whether we are actively caring for someone with Alzheimer's or waiting in awareness and readiness to give care, it's imperative to recognize that these exquisitely vulnerable persons with Alzheimer's trust *us*. Into our hands and hearts they *must* commend their fragile beings. People who are afflicted with Alzheimer's have not chosen their situations of frailty, dependence, and declining capacities. We, however, can choose. We can choose our attitudes and our reactions to their ever-changing, ever-increasing needs.

The vulnerability of persons with Alzheimer's is a sacred call to individuals and to society to be trustworthy. To respond appropriately to our call, caregivers and others with authority and power need to learn about, accept, and embrace the realities of living with Alzheimer's. We all need to observe how the realities of this disease are manifesting in each afflicted person, in each afflicted family, and in each afflicted life. This is, indeed, a challenge. It may be, however, the most fulfilling and rewarding challenge we will ever face.

Into our hands these dear ones with Alzheimer's disease have entrusted the care and cultivation of their fragile beings. May our tender hearts make us compassionate and trustworthy. May our fierce hearts empower us and make us effective.

Spirit-Inspired Caring

"Where does the wind come from Nicodemus?"
"Rabbi, I do not know."
"Nor can you tell where it will go."

"Put yourself into the path of the wind, Nicodemus.
You will be borne along
by something greater than yourself.
You are proud of your position,
content in your security,
but you will perish in such stagnant air.

"Put yourself into the path of the wind, Nicodemus.
Bright leaves will dance before you.
You will find yourself in places you never dreamed of going;
you will be forced into situations
you have dreaded
and find them like a coming home.

"You will have a power you never had before, Nicodemus.
You will be a new man [a new woman].
Put yourself into the path of the wind."

—Myra Scovel

When I moved to Iowa to be with Mom, I understood that making some sacrifices was a part of the decision. I left an established life, including wonderful long-sought, long-prepared-for professional opportunities. I still feel sad, sometimes, when I consider what I left behind. Additionally, there have been and continue to be some undesirable consequences for me. Yet, I have no regrets. My decision to move was the right decision for Mom. And it was the right decision for me; of this I feel certain.

During my decision-making process, and my relocation and transition, I carried the poem *The Wind of the Spirit* close to my heart. This poem first became a guiding light for me in 2003 while I was seeking wisdom about shifting the focus of my ministry to spiritual direction.

I later discovered, quite by accident, that the poet, Myra Scovel, was the mother of my colleague, Rev. Carl Scovel. Ultimately, the truth of this poem guided my decision to care for my mother when Alzheimer's struck; it also chronicled the outcome of my "yes." As Myra's poem predicted, by putting myself into "the path of the wind," I found myself living in Dubuque, Iowa—a hometown I had *never* dreamed of returning to. And I was drawn into a situation that I had previously dreaded: caring for a dependent, vulnerable mother who hadn't protected or cared for me when I was dependent and vulnerable. But this never-dreamed-of, dreaded circumstance surprisingly became a "coming home." When I began this journey, I never dreamed that a nursing home filled with people in various stages of Alzheimer's would become a holy land or that words like *suffering, Alzheimer's, gratitude, meaning,* and *joy* would be spoken in the same sentence, flowing sincerely from my healing heart.

Into the path of the wind . . .

Points of Surrender

After Mom moved to the nursing home and while I still lived in Boston, I was in regular contact with her by phone. She didn't talk much by this time, but the nurses told me she listened attentively, and hearing my voice brought an ear-to-ear smile across her face. One day she found the words to clearly blurt into the phone, "I miss my house!" I sighed, took a breath, and replied, "I know you do, Mom. I know you do." One of Mom's friends had called me to tell me of a visit with her. When the friend tried to leave, Mom clung to her, sobbing, and begged to be taken home.

It seemed to me that Mom was experiencing what Jesus scholar Marcus Borg calls "life in exile." She was separated "from all that was familiar and dear," and now, on the margins of society, felt the depth of her powerlessness. Borg writes that "the feeling of being separated from home and longing for home runs deeply within us . . . and life in exile is marked by deep sadness and an aching loneliness."[1] The solution to exile is, of course, "a journey of return . . . a homecoming." For Mom, there was to be no going home to her house. My coming home brought Mom into connection with a familiar and dear person, and helped us both journey "home" to a "place where God was present."[2]

For many persons with Alzheimer's, nursing homes eventually become a necessity. My mom was vehemently opposed to this idea. She had communicated this to me clearly through her volatile reaction to my proposed plan to visit an adult day center, and her reference to nursing home living as being "garaged." It was heartbreaking to hear how much Mom missed her house and wanted to return to her home of sixty years. This reality, however, is an important point of surrender that Alzheimer's family caregivers often must face. Although many of us have promised our loved ones that we will not move them to nursing homes "no matter what," although we fear they may die shortly after moving to a care facility, and although other family members may condemn us for this choice, Alzheimer's often presents circumstances we can't foresee and can't manage in our homes. In the presence of these circumstances, "no matter what" is overwhelmed by the power of Alzheimer's.

As Sam Keen explored the sacred relationship between love and care in American society, he noticed that we have "transferred as much as possible our responsibility for care to the 'caring professionals,'" whom he refers to as "care-sellers."[3] Keen's observation regarding the transfer of care from homes to facilities is accurate. But in many cases, necessity, rather than the desire to transfer responsibility, is the motivation. His chilling reference to care-sellers, however, makes the necessary surrender to this choice feel even more difficult for families. When caregivers come to this point of surrender, it's important to be empathetic to our loved ones' resistance, understand their feelings of separation and exile, seek guidance and support in facilitating this lifestyle change, and practice forgiving ourselves for not being more than we are and not doing more than we can.

One eighty-something woman put herself in jeopardy because she didn't realize the enormous emotional stress and physical strain she would encounter while trying to care for her husband with Alzheimer's at home. I met Georgia at the nursing home, and she told me of her reluctance to move Roger into a care facility. She had surrendered only after Roger had fallen on top of her. He weighed 250 pounds, and she was a fragile 105 pounds. The fall had broken her arm, which was a lucky outcome because she could have been killed. All caregivers must be prepared to ask for and accept help.

Adult children who want their parents to live with them might work outside the home and therefore be unable to provide the kind of care, attention, socialization, and supervision needed by persons with Alzheimer's, especially as the disease progresses. In these circumstances, home care and adult day programs can offer support for those who can afford it, and the surrender to nursing home care can be delayed.

The ability to afford twenty-four-hour in-home care still might not be a match for the power of Alzheimer's. Two of my friends attempted to keep their moms living independently in their moms' homes. Both found it to be a highly stressful challenge: hiring and keeping track of personnel, making sure all shifts were covered, making sure the care was appropriate, figuring out what to do if an aide couldn't make it because of illness or weather. A friend who lived in New England heard a story about a woman with Alzheimer's who, on a day her home health aide hadn't come, wandered outside, slipped on the ice, and froze to death. Within a week, he had moved his own mother to an assisted living facility.

The aging "industry"—including adult day programs, assisted living facilities, and nursing homes—is growing rapidly to meet the needs of our aging population, particularly those of persons with Alzheimer's, which are the most demanding and daunting. The facilities are unquestionably a personal and social necessity.

For various reasons, some family members do what my mom feared, and so horrifically referred to as "garaging." They drop their loved ones off at care facilities and wash their hands of any further responsibility. Some of them, exhausted by their previous caregiving endeavors, feel relieved that others can take over. Unfortunately, many family members never return. Ever. This absence of family engagement with the residents and staff of nursing homes is another heartbreaking reality of Alzheimer's disease. At this point, persons with Alzheimer's must surrender and adjust since their power to change anything about this reality has vanished.

When people learned that I had moved from Boston to be with Mom, some thought I had made a great sacrifice. Others were unimpressed with my commitment to care for her, citing the freedom I had in my life. Apparently I wasn't shifting my priorities in ways that seemed meaningful to them. It's true that I wasn't a member of the "sandwich generation." I didn't have children or a spouse who needed my attention at the same time I was caring for Mom. My life, however, was complicated in other practical ways: health considerations, the need to relocate across the country, disrupted living situations, doctoral studies, financial pressures, and demanding work.

Caregivers who shared their experiences with me also had complicated practicalities in the context of their busy lives. Mary Anne and Coleen were sandwiched between meeting the needs of their mothers with Alzheimer's, their young children, and their spouses, all while working full-time. Coleen even returned to college and got her bachelor's degree in business during this time. Carl and Steve were sandwiched between caregiving for their moms and their families in addition to the demanding work of parish ministry, which requires meeting the pastoral needs of hundreds of parishioners.

Although our complications were different, we had one thing in common: None of us considered caregiving for our mothers as optional. It became something we *would* do. Along with Arthur Kleinman, it was something we had to do. We organized our lives around this priority, set up schedules, and stuck to them. When a person's needs or a specific activity can't be optional, we human beings always seem to figure out a way to make time and energy for it. This figuring out process ultimately requires us to surrender to the reality that this need can't be changed and to be willing to rearrange our priorities.

Changing priorities is something parents do all the time—often automatically, usually willingly, and sometimes joyfully. Later in life, however, we don't expect to have to make radical changes in our priorities or our patterns to care for our parents or spouses. Alzheimer's disease is shaking up old patterns, though, and inviting us to change our individual and social priorities and respond to the changing realities of need.

In order to integrate Alzheimer's caregiving into an already over-busy life, it could help to think of it as a spiritual practice or discipline. To factor any spiritual practice into our lives, this is how to begin: We develop a practice to which we can willingly and realistically commit; then we make the practice a priority by choosing to do it no matter what. In order to do this, something else will most likely have to be given up. Mary Anne, Coleen, Carl, Steve, and I committed to caregiving in this way, and caregiving became a regular part of our life routines.

Choosing to make our not-easy caregiving roles a priority requires a profound shift, in our attitudes and in our actions. At first it may seem impossible, but with practice, it becomes doable. As with any spiritual practice, we all struggle at the beginning because it's truly an effort to integrate a new priority and routine into our lives. Developing a regular schedule works best. For example, visit Monday through Friday at lunchtime; or Sundays for lunch; or Saturday mornings while doing errands; or on the way home from work on weekdays; or Monday, Wednesday, and Friday for dinner; or Tuesday for dinner and a walk. The important first step in succeeding with any spiritual practice is choosing a schedule that can be maintained.

When I first arrived in Iowa, my friend and spiritual direction colleague, Sister Mary Owen, helped to guide me through my process of shifting and surrendering. Mary Owen was a nurse and had spent a large part of her ministry in nursing homes. Coaching me, she said, "In order to really appreciate what elders in decline have to teach us, we need to go close enough and stay long enough to see their beauty and value." Once we can see, once the spiritual practice of caregiving becomes part of our lives, caregivers may be surprised by unexpected moments of gladness and a deep sense of satisfaction.

Some family members and friends of persons with Alzheimer's will have the best intentions to visit their loved ones regularly. Unfortunately, our best intentions are often met with emotional complications, which are perhaps the greatest deterrent to active caregiving. One resident in Mom's nursing home told me that her only daughter didn't come to visit because she "couldn't stand" seeing people in wheelchairs. Many other family members told me they don't visit because it's just "too hard" for them to see their loved ones in a diminished capacity. It's not because they don't care. It's because it stirs up uncomfortable thoughts and feelings—emotional complications—that most of us don't know how to endure. It's truly terrifying to see the possibilities that life might have in store for us. Everyone, including every resident, knows that nursing homes are usually the last stop before death. No one wants to think about that. I understand. But I also know that emotional complications, once addressed, can be overcome.

One evening, as I walked the two blocks from my new Dubuque home to the nursing home where Mom lived, I was surprised to notice a bounce in my step. My heart felt light and open and joyful. I hadn't felt like this earlier in the day. "Why now?" I wondered. By the time I arrived at the door to the nursing home, my joy was bursting out all over.

Recognizing that joyful anticipation is not the universal response to visiting relatives, friends, and loved ones in nursing homes, I had to reflect a bit to understand why I felt this way. I realized that spending time with Mom and others with Alzheimer's was a pleasure and a relief, because they are people without pretense. Their spontaneous authenticity refreshed me. They always seemed happy to see me, and without having any perceptible expectations of me, they graciously and gratefully received whatever attention and kindness I was able to offer on any given day. I realized that, having come close enough and stayed long enough, I was now recognizing value and beauty in their presence.

Lightness, openness, and joy were not always my responses to nursing homes or to persons with Alzheimer's. When Aunt Maggie had Alzheimer's, she lived in a care facility for fifteen years until she died in 1989. On one hometown visit during my early adulthood, Mom convinced me to accompany her on her weekly visit with her sister. My dearest aunt did not recognize me. Her bulging eyes were blank and her hands clutched a baby doll. She was leaning over her wheelchair, drooling. The unintelligible, garbled noises she made finally drove me from the nursing home to the car, where I waited for Mom—feeling traumatized. As we rode home in silence, I was surprised that she didn't criticize my reactivity or my abrupt departure. We never talked about it, but I had the impression that she understood. She never asked me to go again.

I wasn't drawn back into nursing homes until 2004, when Mom's disease was progressing to the point that she would eventually need constant skilled care. Over the next two years, I visited a number of nursing homes with Alzheimer's units both in Massachusetts, where I lived at the time, and in Iowa, where Mom lived. My tour of one beautiful state-of-the-art facility specializing in Alzheimer's care for persons in various stages of the disease took place during the activities time, which involved ball playing. More than twenty residents sat in a circle in chairs and wheelchairs. Some were leaning and drooling and garbling words. Some clutched dolls or teddy bears. A staff member stood in the center of the circle, throwing a large soft ball to each resident, who then did his or her best to bat it, or catch and throw it, back to the staff member.

It's humbling to admit that my initial internal responses to the nursing home environment were not much different than they had been when I tried to visit Aunt Maggie twenty-five years earlier, although my external composure was more restrained. I didn't bolt out of the facility in a traumatized state. After witnessing the ball-playing scene, however, I did make a hasty, albeit slightly more gracious, exit.

After I assisted Mom with her dinner, we would usually go for a walk together. During nice weather, we walked outside, but on cold, rainy evenings, we walked the long corridors of the nursing home, four hallways on each of three floors. As we passed by the rooms, I often glanced in, mostly looking for decorating ideas for Mom's room. Sometimes I would see residents in their rooms. Occasionally, seeing them would awaken me to the idea that some day I could be in one of those rooms. This possibility frightened me, and I would go home on those nights and weep—for Mom, for the other residents, and for my future lonely, frightened self.

In the midst of these recurring times of lament, I prayed for the strength to embrace my own emotions. Sometimes, from within the fury of my fear, I would hear echoes of encouragement from my friend and caregiving companion, Mary Anne. She had heard the myriad of reasons people offered for not visiting nursing home residents, many from her own siblings. In response, her eternal hopefulness and her clarity of need shone through. She hopes that, when caregivers' hearts are fearful, we will be able to overcome our resistance and be there for our loved ones with Alzheimer's—because they need us. During the times when my practical and emotional complications made the world of Alzheimer's feel impossible for me to touch, I turned to a poem by Sufi mystic Shams al-Din Hafiz for comfort and strength:

> Don't surrender your loneliness
> So quickly.
> Let it cut more deep.
>
> Let it ferment and season you
> As few human
> Or even divine ingredients can.
>
> Something missing in my heart tonight
> Has made my eyes so soft,
> My voice
> So tender,
>
> My need of God
> Absolutely
> Clear.[4]

Each time I encountered the roadblock called fear, I asked for inner and outer help to get beyond it. And I did. Each time I was tempted to turn away, I intentionally worked to shift my attention to Mom and her needs. Although it was productive to recognize and acknowledge my feelings of fear, helplessness, and despair, it wasn't especially comfortable. After consciously meeting and accepting as valid every one of my painful or fearful emotions, however, I was always able to return to the nursing home the next day, always filled with joy on my mission to care for Mom. My teacher, Janet Ramsey, would describe my process and my ability to "bounce back" as "spiritual resiliency."

She believes our ability to be resilient can increase with practice, and that possessing this ability becomes more important as we age and our losses accumulate.[5]

On the evening that my feelings of lightness, openness, and joy caught my attention, I was on my way to lead the ball game for the residents on Mom's floor. No longer running away in fright, I had become the person tossing the ball to drooling, leaning, word-garbling, doll-clutching, smiling, grateful people in various stages of Alzheimer's. I was the joy-filled person in the center of the circle, calling out their names and connecting with each person through eye contact, gentle touch, smiles, and laughter. These people were no longer nursing home residents to me. They had become individuals with names and personalities, with likes and dislikes, with abilities and disabilities, with joys and sorrows, and with families—some who visited and brought joy to the residents and some who didn't visit until death was imminent. Many of the residents had become friends and were part of my daily life. They were friends with life histories (whether or not they could tell me about their histories, their histories existed and informed their interactions). They were friends who possessed the potential to love me and to teach me about living—and dying. There is a Buddhist proverb, "When the student is ready, the teacher appears." These blessed, darling, vulnerable, wise people with Alzheimer's, many of whom had been cast aside like unwanted orphans, had become my important companions and teachers.

Psychiatrist James Gordon explains that we often don't feel the "need to be aware when all is going well," and "life is on kind of an automatic pilot."[6] Without our approval, a diagnosis of Alzheimer's disrupts our patterns and turns our habitual momentum inside out, giving us an opportunity—a mandate perhaps—to shift away from automatic pilot and to wake up. During my journey with Mom through Alzheimer's, I came to understand that waking up is one kind of challenge. Staying awake is another. The message about wakefulness written by thirteenth-century Sufi mystic Rumi often came into my consciousness in response to the stress, pain, and fear entangled in the hearts of those giving care for persons with Alzheimer's disease: "The breeze at dawn has secrets to tell you, don't go back to sleep."[7] Because I trust that there are life-giving secrets within every aspect of life, I knew I needed to stay awake—to all aspects of Alzheimer's, including my uncomfortable feelings— in order to find the hidden secrets.

Family members of nursing home residents with Alzheimer's from all across the country have explained to me that they don't visit more often because seeing the conditions and the care their loved ones receive causes them to feel distressed and helpless. As I weighed the pros and cons about moving to be with Mom, my friend, a nurse in a veterans' nursing facility, warned me that, because of limited time and staff, residents who have family members looking out for them receive more attention and ultimately better care. The overworked and sometimes undertrained certified nursing aides—whose numbers continue to be threatened by Medicare and Medicaid cuts—have been known to forget or neglect their required responsibilities while caring for our loved ones. This can happen in even the best care facilities. Family members have reported finding their loved ones in undignified situations, painful positions, hungry and thirsty, sitting in soiled clothing, and suffering from medication side effects that the nursing staff didn't notice. After witnessing such neglect, some family members have been so upset that they hesitated to return. If they filtered through the emotional storm called "upset," it's likely they would find feelings of helplessness at the core. After making similar discoveries in regard to Mom, I discussed my concerns with nursing home staff. Sometimes I felt heard, sometimes not. Occasionally things improved.

After all of these conversations, however, I usually felt helpless to make any meaningful changes in Mom's life. It's not just in the nursing home setting that Alzheimer's caregivers will feel helplessness—it's a recurrent feeling throughout all the stages of our journeys with our loved ones.

One of my greatest challenges in caring for Mom was trying to ensure that the nursing home delivered the care they had recommended and promised. What they called a "care plan," I interpreted as a sacred covenant to care for my vulnerable mother. In the beginning, I fretted over the details of this plan. I lost sleep worrying that Mom's head wouldn't be elevated to the proper angle when a substitute aide put her to bed and that she would choke during the night. Even though I knew that there was no way to beat death, I did not want my mother to die from this kind of oversight. I also knew that I couldn't possibly monitor the nursing home care twenty-four hours a day.

In the midst of this worry, the thinking of Jewish theologian Abraham Joshua Heschel brought me awareness and comfort. According to Heschel, there are two ways of knowing reality: reason and wonder. Through reason, he explains, we try to make the world conform to our existing concepts of how things should be. In my mind, the nursing home should be implementing—to perfection—every aspect of Mom's care plan. After all, they developed the plan. This reasonable expectation, however, had the potential to create great misery. Because I saw this misery manifested in other nursing home families who relentlessly demanded perfection from the staff, I carefully attended to Heschel's thoughts about wonder. Through wonder we seek to adjust to our world, to pursue authentic awareness of that which is. Wonder requires letting go—staying still until the truth can reveal itself. My worry about Mom's care eventually evolved into a grace-filled surrender. I accepted that many things in the nursing home, everything about Alzheimer's disease, and the time and circumstances of my mother's death were beyond my control. I was face-to-face with what theologian Richard Rohr refers to as the "spirituality of imperfection." I knew the limits of my power and admitted to all that I couldn't change, fix, or make into what I wanted it to be. When we become aware of and surrender to our own powerlessness, according to Rohr, we have to transform. "Great healing," he said, "is always about transforming."[8]

Ultimately, my daily view of the monumental task of caring for the flood of elders, particularly those with dementia, flowing into Mom's nursing home led me to feel admiration for the facility's mission. I matured into a greater understanding of their strengths and limitations, as well as an acceptance of their imperfections, identifying what could and could not be changed.

My surrender to the limits of nursing home care, however, did not in any way lead me to conclude that Mom, or any person with Alzheimer's, is undeserving of better, more informed, more compassionate, and more enlightened care than many are currently receiving. About this, I retained and manifested the courage to speak. One issue that I raised repeatedly was finally investigated, and a facility-wide problem with the computer charting process was discovered. So by raising this issue, I brought about reform within the nursing home and perhaps improvement in the lives of other residents, as well as in Mom's.

The Alzheimer's Association and others, including authors Joanne Koenig Coste and Marty Richards, in her book, *Caresharing*, have introduced the word *carepartners* into the practice of Alzheimer's care. Their common intention, by coining this term, is to emphasize the reciprocity of love and care that flows between persons with Alzheimer's and their families, friends, and communities. To believe that our relationships with persons with Alzheimer's are about more than their neediness and our giving them care requires a shift in attitude about and understanding of Alzheimer's. The purpose of introducing the word *carepartners* into our vocabulary is to empower persons with Alzheimer's and to inform families and friends that persons with Alzheimer's remain an integral and contributing part of our relationships. Considering each other partners in caring speaks to the covenantal relationship of givers and receivers. When this shift in attitude happens, caregivers may feel less burdened, and persons with Alzheimer's may feel more valued.[9]

When I was visiting Mom during the summer of 2004, I experienced reciprocity of care that enlightened me about the carepartner relationship. Shortly after my arrival, I noticed scratchiness in my throat, the usual beginning of an allergic reaction. Later that day, I had a sore throat and mentioned it to Mom when I suggested that we have tea together. The next morning, when I was making breakfast, I saw a bottle of aspirin at my place at the table. Still trying to get a handle on what kind of medication Mom was taking, I asked her, "What's the aspirin for?" She replied, "It's for you. You said you had a sore throat." I was surprised and impressed that she remembered, and so very touched that, through the ravages of Alzheimer's, my Mom still wanted to take care of me. "Oh, yes, Mom, I do. Thank you so much," I said as I hugged her. Without taking the aspirin, or any other medical intervention, my sore throat went away quickly, and the anticipated allergic reaction didn't happen. Perhaps Mom's exemplary effort at carepartnering had stimulated my immune system enough to heal me.

After Mom moved to the nursing home, I expanded my understanding of carepartnering to include the staff. The nursing home provided Mom with her basic needs: shelter and food, baths and toileting, appropriate furniture and linens, laundry services, and assistance with the tasks of daily living. I provided her with clothing, companionship, more assistance with the activities of daily living, attention, fun, and love. The nursing home scheduled activities and outings; I accompanied Mom to the activities and on the outings, helping her to participate in and enjoy them. As the structure of the nursing home evolved to include more state-of-the-art care for dementia residents, I was able to select the nursing aides I wanted to work with Mom. I chose aides who were mature, devoted to elder care, and seemed to have naturally developed a friendship with her. They were especially kind to her and attentive to the details of her care plan. They helped her maintain her capabilities, such as walking, and encouraged her to continue to grow. These aides and I communicated well, and they kept me informed about Mom's accomplishments and any changes in her habits and behavior. We were Mom's eyes, recognizing what she needed; and we were Mom's voice, keeping each other informed of her ever-changing abilities and needs. I came to truly feel that the nursing home and I were in a cooperative carepartnership for Mom, each of us providing what the other could not.

In spite of her increasing limitations, Mom continued to demonstrate her desire to care for me. In the evenings, an aide would help her stand up from her wheelchair. Once she was standing, we hugged. I put my arms around her and she put her arms around me. She held me so tightly that it could only be described as holding me like she would never let me go. Sometimes we swayed to music, but mostly we just stood and hugged, and I would scratch her back. I know Mom loved this time for hugging, because she always had a broad smile and an ecstatic look on her face. She also made a purring sound. At this stage of her illness, her fingers were constricted and her hands almost constantly curled into a fist. Often while I was scratching her back, I could feel her fingers uncurling and ever so slightly moving back and forth. She was trying to scratch my back while I scratched hers. Mom could barely move any part of her body voluntarily, and yet she was making a clear effort to be my carepartner. She was trying to give me the same kind of physical pleasure and comfort I was giving her. Her efforts moved me deeply.

Mom's desire to be an active carepartner reached beyond me to the staff who cared for her with love and devotion. Alexis, her primary aide on the afternoon-evening shift, had a unique gift for interacting with people with dementia. Maybe it was the tone of her voice or the encouragement on her face, but something about Alexis brought out impressive responsiveness. Mom and Alexis became close.

One night, however, Mom caused Alexis a moment of worry. Toward the end of her life, when her hands were curled, Mom's grip became viselike. To get her to let go of something, we often had to pry open her fingers, gently of course. On this night, Alexis was crouched on the floor in front of Mom's wheelchair, putting on her shoes. Slowly, Mom reached out her arm and put her hand on top of Alexi's head. Alexis was afraid that Mom was going to grab her hair and not let go. Then she would be stuck there, probably in hair-pulling pain, until someone happened by to rescue her. But Mom didn't grab Alexis's hair. She very gently stroked the top of her head, just as I had stroked and massaged Mom's. Mom was making an effort to give Alexis the same kind of comfort and pleasure she had received from me.

Once caregivers can shift their attitudes away from the presumed solitariness of their role and open their hearts to include the possibility of carepartnering, there is ample opportunity for everyone in the partnership to experience healing.

A colleague recently mentioned how much she hates the word *surrender*. This is understandable. In our culture, *surrender* is most often used in the context of warfare and carries a connotation of defeat or failure. In the context of the spiritual journey, however, surrender is an acknowledgment and ultimately an acceptance of reality. Some might be more comfortable with the Buddhist notion of *detachment*. Others might prefer the less emotionally charged phrase *letting go*. But *surrender*—defined by Webster's as "to give oneself up, as into the power of another"—

seems to best describe both the requirement and the gift for carepartners on the spiritual journey through Alzheimer's. As their brains deteriorate, persons with Alzheimer's will naturally, gracefully evolve into surrender. This disease is asking caregivers not for combat but for cooperation.

The power of Alzheimer's is still so great that, for now, only surrender will bring us spiritual victory and peace of mind and heart.

The Dance of Yes and No

There's a dance that happens in all of our lives in between yes and no. It's a dance of discernment and choice as old as recorded history. In the book of Deuteronomy in the Hebrew scriptures, God speaks to Moses about this dance: "I call heaven and earth to witness against you today that I have set before you life and death, blessings and curses. Choose life so that you and your descendants may live."[10]

The guidance in this passage is clear, but which choice is the life-giving one might not be. If we choose to say yes to someone or something, it usually means we're choosing to say no to someone or something else. As we're defining and choosing our attitudes, priorities, and practices in relationship to caring for someone with Alzheimer's disease, this dance between yes and no will often be in full swing.

The intricacies of the dance became clear for me when I read the thought-provoking work of Richard Foster, Quaker author and theologian. In his introduction to Thomas Kelly's *A Testament of Devotion*, Foster recalls the exact words in Kelly's book that resonated with his soul and facilitated a personal transformation: "'We feel honestly the pull of many obligations and try to fulfill them all. And we are unhappy, uneasy, strained, oppressed, and fearful we shall be shallow.'" And then Foster read the words that brought him hope: "We have hints that there is a way of life vastly richer and deeper than all this hurried experience...We have seen and know some people who seem to have found this deep Center of living, where the fretful calls of life are integrated, where no as well as yes can be said with confidence."[11]

Kelly's certainty that some people have found a divine center of living that supports their ability to confidently say no as well as yes shook up Foster, because the ability was foreign to him. He could easily say yes, because doing so usually supported his "egoistic view" of himself as spiritual and self-sacrificing. He worried, however, what others would think of him if he said no. Right then and there—in the midst of chaos at bustling Dulles International Airport, where Foster first read *A Testament of Devotion*—he paused and prayed for "the ability to say no when it was right and good."[12]

Very soon, Foster was invited into the dance. Shortly after returning home from his travels, a denominational executive presented him with an enticing professional opportunity scheduled on the same night he had planned to spend time with his family. Foster said no to the denominational executive and yes to keeping his commitment to be with his family. He describes the result of this choice as "electrifying." "I had yielded to the Center....That simple no coming out of divine promptings set me free from the tyranny of others. Even more, it set me free from my own inner clamoring for attention and recognition and applause."[13]

In humility, Foster then writes about his embarrassment that such a small and seemingly insignificant incident facilitated such an important inner transformation. "But there it is, a trivial event, yet it changed everything for me.... At least I know that often the genuinely significant issues are decided in the small corners of life."[14]

Jewish theologian, Martin Buber, reminds us often to hallow (make holy) the every day. According to Buber, "Hallowing transforms [our] urges by confronting them with holiness and making them *responsible* toward what is holy."[15] Buber further explains that this transformation from life-draining automatic responses to life-giving, "holy" choices does not happen inside a solitary individual. According to Buber, our transformations can only be manifested *in relation*.

In the Christian New Testament, we find an example of how "Yes," spoken in relation, manifests healing and transformation. Matthew 15:21-28 tells the story of a Canaanite woman who comes out of the crowd, shouting at Jesus to "have mercy on me . . . my daughter is tormented by a demon." Of all the healing stories in the New Testament, this one stands out, because it tells of Jesus being transformed by a true encounter with another person.

Disturbed by the woman's persistence, the disciples urge Jesus to send her away. Jesus explains to the woman that he has been "sent only to the lost sheep of Israel." The woman then presents herself to Jesus from the deep center of living, revealing her bravery, her humility, and her dignity. She kneels before him, saying, "Lord help me." Jesus, however, remains unmoved and continues to say no. Finally, in response to her plaintive cries for help, he explains, "It is not fair to take the children's food and throw it to the dogs."

The woman again speaks words from her divine promptings. Through meditation on this passage, I began to see her words in the context of the improvisational theater practice of yes/and:

"Yes, Lord, yet . . ." she begins. It is this yes, this acceptance of Jesus's explanation, that facilitates a transformation for Jesus and the healing of the woman's daughter. Unlike the Pharisees, who are always arguing with Jesus, challenging him and pushing him into defending his argument and maintaining his power position of teacher or prophet in order for his point to be received, the woman simply accepts and agrees with Jesus's position. She says, "Yes, Lord." She shows her respect and understanding; then she offers her perspective: ". . . yet, even the dogs eat the crumbs that fall from their masters' table." The courage and humility of her earlier actions and pleas have not opened Jesus' heart, but the yes that flows from her center opens first his mind—because she has acknowledged what he said as valid—and then his heart. From this place of openness, he chooses to step into what Buber calls "direct relation"[16] with her. He chooses to override his bias toward healing only the Israelites. From his divine center, Jesus says no to his previous limited understanding of his mission; and he says yes to the radical choice to heal a Canaanite. "Woman, great is your faith! Let it be done for you as you wish." And her daughter is healed instantly.[17]

The yes/and practice of improvisational theater requires that we have first learned to validate and accept the offer by saying yes. The practice then invites us to *advance the offer* by saying "and. . . ." We then have the opportunity to add our own inspired truth (or inspired fiblette if necessary). Choosing this life-affirming response often encourages a connection to flourish. The opposite step in the dance is to *block the offer* by saying no, denying the other, and/or arguing and creating a struggle for power and control.

Inspired by Foster, the Canaanite woman, and Jesus, I carried their examples of saying yes and no from the divine center into the nursing home and into every interaction I had with Mom and her neighbors. In the place that Mom referred to as a garage, with people in the midst of cognitive decline, I looked for opportunities to hallow the everyday experiences of life with Alzheimer's disease. Repeatedly, I was offered life or death, blessings or curses. I consciously tried to choose life and blessings.

Because of my school schedule, Mom had been living in the nursing home for four months before I was able to travel to Iowa during my winter break to see her. Those first days I spent with her turned out to be about much more than visiting. Those days, and all the years that followed, became an immersion experience in Alzheimer's reality and care, providing limitless practice in the life-changing dance of yes and no.

Throughout Mom's first months at the nursing home, the distressing departure episodes—including clinging, begging to be taken home, angry outbursts, and crying—had continued. Every time someone visited Mom and left her, there was an emotional scene. My desire to help her avoid this upsetting experience became my first lesson in saying no when it was right and good. I was surprised to discover that, in order to say yes to what Mom needed, I had to say no to myself, to my beliefs and habits about what constituted a proper good-bye.

When it was time for me to say good-bye to someone who had visited, my habit was to walk with the visitor to the door, to express gratitude for the visit, and to say good-bye with a physical gesture, a kiss, hug, or touch. I learned this habit from my gracious mother. However, this very habit of acknowledging our time together, expressing gratitude, and sharing a physical connection now caused turmoil for Mom. She didn't want her visitors to leave without her; she didn't want the connection to be broken by good-bye. Accepting where Mom was in the disease process and accepting her ever-changing needs were the places where I needed to express my yes.

As the time approached for me to leave, I told Mom that soon I would have to go for a while. I told her where I was going (to have lunch and a rest), and when I would be back (5:30, in time to have dinner with her). When it was the actual time for me to leave, however, I made sure Mom was occupied in other ways. The first time I tried this was after lunch. We waited together in Mom's room for the aide to come and help her to the rest room. When the aide arrived, Mom and I walked across her room. She looked happy walking with me as we held hands. When we reached the aide, I gave Mom's hand to her. As soon as they made eye contact, Mom was fully engaged with the aide. They walked away from me and into the rest room together. Mom never looked back. There was no distress for her in this process of my leave-taking. The aide told me there was no emotional upset. Instead, Mom napped away the afternoon in a happy glow from our time together. Her happiness was still glowing when I returned at 5:30.

On other days when it was time for me to leave, I waited until Mom had dozed off in her chair, or I arranged to stay until she was walking with someone else to meals or on her way to the bath. From the first day of my first visit with Mom until the day she died, it was always hard for me to leave her. But by being aware of timing, Mom's schedule, and her attentiveness to other people, things, and activities, I could make sure that the separation was not stressful for her. Although it was a less than satisfying good-bye for me, and at times required me to stay a bit longer than I had planned, the choice was right and good for Mom.

My experiences with Mom during the early and middle stages of Alzheimer's, reading *Learning to Speak Alzheimer's*, my conversations with the psychiatrist and the improv teacher, and the possibilities for healing and transformation I discovered in my spiritual reading—all had solidified for me the critical importance of acceptance in the presence of Alzheimer's disease. Reinforcing my learning, a friend shared a fascinating research study on stress-related disorders among dementia caregivers. This study determined that acceptance is the only coping technique shown to effectively reduce caregiver stress.[18] This knowledge motivated me to fully accept the ever-changing landscape and the challenges of Alzheimer's. It wasn't easy, but integrating improvisation with my spiritual practices helped me to accept what was and then notice what was possible. Acceptance became a way of saying yes to Mom as well as to my own well-being.

After I moved to Iowa and gained more in-depth knowledge and experience from interactions with persons with Alzheimer's and their caregivers, my understanding of saying yes in the context of Alzheimer's care became more refined. I discovered that saying yes doesn't actually translate into a literal yes, which could have catastrophic consequences. One woman I met at a dementia care conference told me that her husband wanted to take his lawn chair into the middle of the lake. In improv class, that desire could initiate an entertaining scene. In real life, though, it's dangerous and not something to agree with or to approve. In order to avoid conflict in that situation, some creative, compassionate improvising would be necessary. Since it's highly possible that he didn't realize the lake was made of water and couldn't be walked on, one initial intervention could be to tell him he will sink and to show him the water is not solid by splashing. Keeping him safe would be the priority, but inquiring about his need and what he was trying to accomplish by taking the lawn chair into the lake, and then offering alternatives, would lead to the most healing solution.

I learned that saying yes in the context of Alzheimer's is not necessarily about agreement or approval. It's about adopting an attitude of acceptance and affirmation. Figuring out what was happening for Mom—what she was feeling and what she needed—was, at times, like a five-star puzzle, often bringing me face-to-face with that dreaded feeling of helplessness. But accepting her, affirming her, and guarding her self-esteem were my goals, and so I puzzled on.

Reality orientation, which many caregivers still try to implement with persons with dementia, is the opposite of acceptance and affirmation. Reality orientation is about changing people and correcting people. Being constantly corrected is annoying and demeaning for anyone. I don't like it, and I'm sure persons with Alzheimer's don't like it either. Unfortunately, I heard endless corrections happening in the nursing home on a daily basis.

"No. This isn't your milk." "No, you can't go in there. It's not your room." "No. I don't work on Friday. I work on Monday. How many times do I have to remind you?" "Oh, no. This is not your husband. Stay away from him. You're bothering him." "You can't take that. It's not yours." These negations and corrections were issued relentlessly, presumably with good intentions. Perhaps those offering the corrections thought they would make some kind of lasting difference as they might with children, who will remember and learn from the stated boundaries.

As I sat with Mom in the resident lounge, assisted her with her meals in the dining room, and walked with her through the nursing home corridors, my ears were constantly barraged by these corrections. Listening to them wore me out and made me feel vicariously annoyed. One day, thinking there had to be another way to interact, I recalled a scene I had witnessed while walking along the beach in Maine. A man was standing at the shoreline while icy waves washed over his feet and ankles. Using his arms to beckon to his daughter who was playing in the waves of deeper water, he called to her, "Honey, come in closer to shore." This sweet invitation brought me to a halt and a moment of awareness. If I had been the parent, concerned for my child's safety, I probably would have done what my parents did—issue a firm order that sounded like this: Don't go out so far!

"Honey, come in closer to shore" versus "Don't go out so far." The energy of the first statement carries a concerned but loving invitation. The second is a correction, carrying with it the clear message that the child has done something wrong.

On two separate days, I witnessed scenes in Mom's nursing home representing these polar opposite messages. And I observed the powerful effect of these differing messages on the feelings and mood of someone with Alzheimer's.

In the nursing home, all of the residents had plastic nameplates that slid into metal brackets attached to the wall next to the doors of their rooms. One day, a darling resident, Regina, appeared in the doorway of the small dining area where the residents with Alzheimer's ate their meals. She had the biggest smile on her face. In her hands was a large stack of nameplates, which she had collected from all the rooms on the floor.

"Oh my, Regina, you've collected the nameplates," remarked Kathy, the regular companion aide assigned to this station. As Kathy, who was a natural yes-sayer, received the nameplates from Regina's hands, her eyes were round with surprise. "I do believe you got them all," she said with a glint of amusement in her voice. "Good job. Thank you."

Regina's smile remained, and she seemed so pleased with herself. She stayed close by Kathy throughout lunch. Later that afternoon, the aide walked around the floor with Regina hand in hand. As they replaced all the nameplates, Regina tried to read the names and was visibly proud of her ability to help reinstall the nameplates.

The next day, Regina again appeared in the doorway of the dining area. Again she had a big smile and her hands full of nameplates. On this day, a substitute aide was working.

"*Oh no*, Regina!" the aide screeched. "These are not yours. You can't do that."

Snatching the nameplates from Regina's hands, shaking her head, and looking very angry, the aide muttered, "Bad. This is very bad."

Regina's smile instantly disappeared and she slouched in despair. She turned around, walked out of the dining area, and went to her room. She spent the rest of the day alone, in bed, refusing meals. Observing these two scenes, I felt Regina's joy and pride on the first day and her sadness and shame on the second day. One aide was affirming. She accepted Regina's offer. The other aide was correcting. She blocked Regina's offer. The correction and the subsequent depression, however, didn't deter Regina from collecting the nameplates in the future.

Persons with Alzheimer's who are being corrected, whose realities are being denied, can become angry. Some will become depressed from repressing their anger, and they will withdraw. Others will strike out verbally if they're still able to talk. Those who are able to voluntarily move their bodies sometimes react with physical force. Theologian and ethicist Stephen Pattison explains that whenever an experience that causes someone to feel ashamed is "bypassed or ignored, rage and aggression [are] likely to occur."[19] Ashamed and angry persons with Alzheimer's can't explain or process their feelings or reactions; but their feelings still exist, and their reactions are very real and valid. If the nursing home staff isn't specifically trained to investigate and interpret these behaviors, residents are often responded to with psychotropic medication to control their "acting out behaviors" rather than with understanding and empathy.

Inspired by the first rule of improvisation, my main intention in my dances of yes and no with Mom and her neighbors was to make them "look good." Instead of reminding them of errors (from my perspective), judging them harshly, negating their reality, or attempting to reorient them into my world, I committed myself to interacting with them in ways that accepted them, affirmed them, made them feel important, and enhanced their sense of worth and dignity. The scenes with Regina brought to life my reading and research. As Professor Earl Thompson points out, "Every interaction we have with others is fraught with the possibility of creating shame or healing pride,"[20] Regina's reactions heightened my awareness of my own words and actions. I became more conscious of my impact on all those around me, especially vulnerable persons with Alzheimer's, who are highly sensitive to emotions and emotional energy. An entire floor of residents could feel upset in various ways from witnessing corrections, negations, and emotional outbursts.

Buber's thinking further informed me about the spiritual

implications of the improvisation practice yes/and in the context of Alzheimer's caregiving. When we affirm persons with Alzheimer's by saying yes to their choices and realities, we are stepping into direct relation with them; we are recognizing and acknowledging their divine essence. Persons with Alzheimer's make their offers to us, and we accept them. "Hence, the relationship means being chosen and choosing." We can co-create affirming and healing experiences (or not) through our choices. This type of relation happens only with our whole beings, and when two whole beings meet, healing can happen. According to Buber, "all real living is meeting."[21]

The yes/and practice enables caregivers to expand their capacity for relating to persons with Alzheimer's, who are almost always presenting themselves to us with their whole beings, their divine essences shining through. It's we who need to reach beyond our habits, conventions, and prejudices, our egos, needs, and judgments to meet them with our whole beings. When we cross over into their worlds and advance the offers they extend to us, we open the door for true meeting, for true healing.

I was leaving the nursing home one night, passing by a group of women residents gathered near the nurses' station. Ellie was there every night when I left, usually slumped over in her wheelchair, asleep. This night, however, she was wide awake and very agitated. As I walked toward her I noticed that she was shaking her clenched fists at me, actually yelling.

"You can't have him!" Ellie shouted.

This was such an impressive scene that I stopped. I leaned down so I was at eye level with Ellie. Looking into her eyes, I accepted her offer when I said, "I can't have him!" I advanced the conversation with curiosity by asking, "Well, why not?"

Ellie's irate response surprised me: "Because we took vows."

When trying to meet persons with Alzheimer's in their world, it's very important to know and play the role you have been cast into. In this interaction, Ellie had cast me into the role of the other woman. I was Jezebel! I got it. But she was still so very upset. In an effort to create a healing moment, I said yes to being Jezebel and yes to making Ellie look good. With these yeses, I made an effort to be responsible to what was holy in life.

In relationship to Ellie, I chose a life-giving response. Looking again into her angry eyes, I said, "You're right, Ellie. I can't have him because he still loves you. I was wrong, and I'm sorry."

As soon as Ellie heard me say this, she calmed down. Her entire body relaxed. She lowered her arms into her lap and her clenched fists opened. Her anger dissipated. Then she replied, "Well, that's very big of you."

I was so surprised by Ellie's gracious words that my only response was a smile and a grateful heart. "Thank you, Ellie," I said. She took my hands, we looked at each other, and we both smiled warmly.

In this meeting with Ellie, which took only a moment of my time, something very profound happened—for Ellie and for me. Ellie calmed down. She had been angry and agitated, but after this interaction, she was calm. This was the observable outcome. Based on what she said, we can speculate that she felt vindicated over a long-ago wound, and possibly some healing happened for her. But what happened for me was remarkable. From Ellie's response to my apology, I felt deeply forgiven—for every bad thing I'd ever done, actually. This meeting with Ellie felt like "real living" to me even though it happened completely in her world, and she thought I was someone else.

By practicing the first rule of improvisation, I was actually manifesting the recommended goal of dementia care described by Tom Kitwood and Kathleen Breden, "to enhance well-being through facilitating a sense of personal worth, a sense of agency, social confidence, and a basic trust or security in the environment and in others."[22] This specific caregiving practice of making my scene partner look good was healing—for Mom, for me, for Regina, for Ellie. Practicing it gave me repeated experiences of what Buber taught and Foster discovered: Transformation happens in the small corners, in the hallowed everyday, from the yes or the no spoken from our deep center of living.

The Present Moment

One of the highlights of my college experience happened by surprise. New friends had convinced me to attend a concert by a relatively unknown folksinger, John Denver. I'd never heard of him but wanted to become friends with the classmates who invited me, so off I went, reluctantly. The concert was astounding, and we all became instant fans. But the highlight came after the concert. While we were having fries and pop at the Bridge restaurant in Dubuque, John Denver came in and we all met him! This moment marked the beginning of a life-long appreciation for his music and admiration for his spiritual and humanitarian evolution.

More than thirty years later, John Denver's song "On the Wings of a Dream" inspired me as I accompanied Mom through Alzheimer's disease. He sang about dreaming and dying, about awakening to the awareness that "the moment at hand is the only thing we really own."[23] Denver's lyrics remind us of a deep, spiritual truth: What's real in every human life is happening right now—in this moment at hand.

Many of us, however, have come to almost worship our happy and important memories. Just as many of us are haunted by memories of painful experiences and can't move forward with our lives in a healthy way. Still others find our joy and pleasure in dreaming about and planning for the future. We expect a new baby. We look forward to a graduation or a wedding or a vacation. We anticipate buying a new car or our first home. Yet many of us feel worry and dread about the unknowns of tomorrow. Still-unidentified challenges lurking around the next corner make us feel nervous and afraid. Whether embedded with joy or sorrow, memories and futures have significance in our lives. In reality, though, our pasts are gone and our tomorrows may never arrive.

Everything that's real in our lives is right here, right now. Sometimes we'd rather forget, deny, or avoid the importance of now, especially when the current experiences of our lives are difficult to embrace. Feelings of loss, grief, anger, abandonment, rejection, fear, loneliness, disappointment, and sadness often send us searching for distractions, of which there are many in our busy lives. If we instead choose to accept the present moment, our hearts, minds, and spirits will awaken to the wisdom of putting the past and the future into perspective. Then we can focus our attention, accordingly, on the right now.

"Do not dwell in the past, do not dream of the future," the Buddha tells us. "Concentrate the mind on the present moment." Ancient and modern theologians and spiritual teachers, poets, musicians, and physicians—many of whom have been my life guides before and during Mom's Alzheimer's diagnosis—have repeated the same message: The present moment is the one that calls for and merits our attention. Now is where we will find reality, connection, meaning, joy, and, ultimately, love. For those seeking to find spiritual meaning on the journey through Alzheimer's, it's important to mention that *this* moment at hand, the only thing we truly own, is most often where we will experience true meetings with ourselves, others, and God.

Real interpersonal communion, according to Martin Buber, begins in between us—person to person. It begins when human beings relate to one another from the position of I to Thou, rather than relating as I to It.[24] When we relate to others as I-It, we consider them as objects, and this always results in separation, loneliness, and disconnection. *Mis-meeting* and *miscounter* are words Buber uses "to designate the failure of a real meeting" between persons.[25]

In a story from his autobiography, *Encounter: Autobiographical Fragments*, Buber described an I-Thou meeting that happened in a childhood moment, while he was petting his beloved horse.

> When I stroked the mighty mane, sometimes marvelously smooth-combed, at other times just as astonishingly wild, and felt the life beneath my hand, it was as though the element of vitality itself bordered on my skin, something that was not I, was certainly not akin to me, palpably the other, not just another, really the Other, itself.[26]

There were no interfering thoughts about the past or the future to distract eleven-year-old Martin. There were no regrets, no worries; there was just now. And in the now, he experienced awareness, presence, and connection. In the fleeting, extraordinary experience of being completely present in that moment, Martin Buber felt life beneath his hand, and he recognized this experience as connection with a transcendent presence.

Gerald May, who became an important influence during my training as a spiritual director, described an experience similar to Buber's. "I can remember experiencing it in childhood, standing in a field and looking at the sky and just *being* in love. . . . It was like being immersed in an atmosphere of love, feeling very alive, very present in the moment, intimately connected with everything around me."[27]

"The deepest level of communication," according to Catholic writer and mystic Thomas Merton, "is not communication but communion. It is beyond words, and it is beyond speech, and it is beyond concept."[28] Merton is not suggesting that we will discover a "new unity" within deep communion. He believed that we are discovering the "older unity," that we are recovering and touching "our original unity."

Often in Mom's presence, I felt Buber's "Other" and May's "being in love." In moments when I brushed Mom's hair or helped her lick an ice-cream cone or watched her fingers remembering how to make music with piano keys, the communion beyond verbal communication described by Merton brought us alive. We transcended time and space. We were together and connected—in the now.

Coleen and I became friends at the nursing home. By the time we met, she had been her mom's faithful companion and advocate on the journey through Alzheimer's for almost ten years. Even after all those years of coming regularly to a nursing home, Coleen still felt particularly alive and connected in the presence of Ilene and others with Alzheimer's. When Coleen came to the nursing home to be with her mother, her eyes saw beyond the sea of wheelchairs and heard beneath the garbled speech. She noticed the hands of residents reaching out to her as she passed by. She recognized humanity in their continuing desire for connection, and she reached back.

A priest-resident of the nursing home, a person with Alzheimer's, sat at the main entrance, greeting visitors and residents coming and going from the building. Coleen greeted him every day when she arrived, and she paused to hold his hand every time she left. "The warmth in his hand made me feel good," she said. "Sometimes when you feel somebody's hand, you can feel God in there. This is a presence that is not taken away by Alzheimer's."

Sometimes these transcendent moments seem to happen mysteriously, opening our entire beings to the presence of a life-giving spirit. These moments, rich with love and presence, are available to us—everywhere, always, in the hallowed everyday experiences. But it's up to us to pause, to be awake and aware, and to open ourselves to receiving them. When we notice and talk about these moments, we often refer to them as peak experiences or moments of grace.

Buber also teaches about the importance of the connection that happens in between us during dialogue, whether in the form of communication or communion. "I have to tell it again and again," he said. "I have no doctrine. I only point out something. I point out reality, I point out something in reality which has not or too little been seen. I take him who listens to me by his hand and lead him to the window. I push open the window and point outside. I have no doctrine, I carry on a dialogue."[29]

Looking through the window at the reality of Alzheimer's, caregivers bear witness to the unpredictable nature of a disease that has no firm doctrine for directing us into understanding. We see that Alzheimer's requires patient, consistent attention to the dialogue which is taking place between caregivers and persons with the disease all the time. Looking through the window, observant caregivers can't help but notice the ability of persons with Alzheimer's to be completely present in the moment. This complete presence is often their contribution to the dialogue. This complete presence is comparable to Buber's pointing finger. Persons with Alzheimer's are doing their best to show us their reality, "which has not or too little been seen."

Persons with Alzheimer's are often, literally, pointing at doors, for which they have a particular fascination. Many will seek to open every closed door they pass. Dr. Allen Power reminds caregivers to pay attention to behaviors that are commonly and repeatedly expressed by persons with Alzheimer's, such as wandering or opening doors. He recommends "curiosity." They are leading us to a window and pointing. But at what? A desire to go home? To be free? To find a loved one? To look at their clothing? To find the kitchen? To go to work? Where do they want to go? What are they looking for? Pointing to? Caregivers need to assume these actions have meaning, and to seek to know and understand what's beneath them.[30]

Dr. Pierre Parenteau chimes in, "It's our responsibility to decode what a patient is trying to tell us through his/her conduct. For instance, if a person starts undressing in a place that seems inappropriate, he/she may be trying to tell us that he/she needs to use the washroom." He recommends "intuition."[31]

Doorknobs often riveted Mom's attention. She would look at the knob, carefully turn it while intently watching it move, pull the door open, push the door closed, then repeat. If allowed, this activity would go on for a long time—perhaps twenty minutes. This kind of focused, in-the-moment door-opening behavior might disturb some caregivers, particularly if it lasts for a long time, but I was both intrigued and delighted whenever Mom did it. At the very least, it seemed to be good exercise for her arm!

During earlier stages of my life journey, medical professionals treating stress-related illnesses and spiritual practitioners teaching the techniques and benefits of meditation and contemplative prayer had been my important teachers. And now, here they were again, offering guidance for the journey through Alzheimer's. These teachers encouraged me to consider twenty minutes of focused attention on anything—a candle flame, a flower, my breath, even a doorknob—as a highly desirable, health-improving, life-changing skill to acquire and to cultivate. Because one benefit of focused attention can be the deepened experiences of life described by Buber, May, and Merton, many intelligent and enlightened beings—past and present—have endeavored to attain this ability. Author Henry Miller understood this: "The moment one gives close attention to anything, even a blade of grass, it becomes a mysterious, awesome, indescribably magnificent world in itself."[32]

A doorknob and a door, and what was on the other side, may have constituted a magnificent world for Mom. As I paid close attention to her opening and closing her closet door, and occasionally reaching slowly and deliberately for the hangers inside, she definitely became an awesome, magnificent world for me.

Through her disease and the process of decline that I witnessed on a daily basis, I came to understand that this moment at hand—this fleeting, precious moment with Mom—was the only moment she had and the only moment we had together. Being able to meet Mom as Thou, even as her capacities diminished, and finding joy with her, was like manna from heaven in the desert of Alzheimer's disease.

In praising the ability of persons with Alzheimer's to focus their attention so completely, it's not my intention to glorify the cognitive decline that is part of Alzheimer's; nor is it my intention to dismiss the sense of loss, confusion, and frustration that family caregivers inevitably experience over their loved ones' forgotten pasts and their unawareness of the future. Alzheimer's, indeed, creates suffering, and it would be cruel to ask loved ones to deny their suffering.

In reaction to the cries of caregivers with "broken hearts and tired lives" (an apt description), Jane Thibault and Richard Morgan ask, "Can we offer any answer, any consolation, any words to sustain the caregivers of parents, spouses, relatives, and friends so that their once-strong bonds of mutual relationship can somehow survive?"[33] By pointing to the ability of persons with Alzheimer's to be in the moment, my intention is to answer the question of Thibault and Morgan with a resounding "Yes." There *are* words, answers, and consolations to offer. In every I-Thou moment, the strong bonds of mutual relationship *can* survive and thrive. Additionally, caregivers are invited to consider another perspective, one that includes the possibility of interpreting the losses and behaviors that are characteristic of Alzheimer's in other ways.

At age thirty-seven, Harvard brain scientist Jill Taylor suffered a massive stroke that left her "so completely disabled," that she described herself "as an infant in a woman's body."[34] Taylor's loss—of language and executive brain functions was similar to losses experienced by persons with Alzheimer's. She describes her experience:

> I met a growing sense of peace. In place of that constant chatter that had attached me to the details of my life, I felt enfolded by a blanket of tranquil euphoria. . . . As the language centers in my left hemisphere grew increasingly silent and I became detached from the memories of my life, I was comforted by an expanding sense of grace. In this void of higher cognition and details pertaining to my normal life, my consciousness soared into an all-knowingness, a "being at one" with the universe. . . . In a compelling sort of way, it felt like the good road home and I liked it.[35]

For the reasons Taylor describes, including "being at one with the universe," the desire (by cognitively intact, intelligent, enlightened persons) to be present in the moment has been demonstrated for thousands of years. Through the practice of meditation and contemplative prayer, spiritual teachers and disciples from every major religious tradition have deliberately sought to experience this state.[36] In the twentieth century, medical practitioners began to recognize that health benefits could be achieved through the focused attention of meditation practice. Decades ago, scientific studies first documented the potential of this practice to reduce stress and improve health.[37] Ongoing studies at Harvard University indicate a correlation between meditation and brain health, including memory retention.[38]

Vipassana, or "insight meditation" (also known as "mindfulness"),[39] is a form of meditation from the Buddhist tradition, and over many years, it has been an enlightening and healing practice for me. The goals of mindfulness meditation are to quiet the mind and body and to be present in the moment, noticing, accepting, and responding to what is, right now. Many people think that meditation can be practiced only when they're sitting on a cushion on the floor in a quiet room, with incense wafting through the space and other meditators chanting *om* or another foreign-sounding mantra. What makes mindfulness a special practice is that it can happen off the cushion in everyday activities. The skills learned through sitting and walking meditation can be applied to everything one does, like eating, washing dishes, brushing teeth, etc. As this skill is developed, one lives increasingly in the present moment and participates more fully in everything he or she does. One Buddhist master who was accomplished in the practice of mindfulness said simply, "When I eat, I eat. When I sleep, I sleep."

The words of the Buddhist master could also be a description of persons with Alzheimer's: When they eat, they eat. When they sing, they sing. When they hug, they hug. When they play ball, they play ball. Buddhist nun Pema Chödrön writes, "If we can experience the moment we're in, we discover that it is unique, precious and completely fresh." This completely fresh moment "never happens twice," she adds. "One can appreciate and celebrate each moment—there's nothing more sacred. There's nothing more vast or absolute. In fact, there's nothing more!"[40]

When we notice that our loved ones with Alzheimer's are intently focused on something, we can consider it an opportunity to pause and join them in the moment, to be fascinated by the magnificent doorknob, drinking fountain, piano keys, or flower—for even a moment. We may be surprised and delighted to discover that we have the potential, right along with our loved ones with Alzheimer's, to lose ourselves and experience a sense of presence, and perhaps even peace.

The benefits of mindfulness don't require a formal sitting meditation practice and they're attainable even within the overwhelming context of Alzheimer's caregiving. Whenever I allowed myself to fully *be* with Mom during her fascination with doorknobs (or with wiping tables, washing dishes, pushing the button on the TV remote and watching the channels change, or turning the drinking fountain on and off), instead of being impatient and wanting to hustle her off to whatever I had planned, I could choose to breathe more deeply and relax. I began to notice details about whatever she was doing—color, texture, and sound, for example—and to experience my feelings of sorrow and joy as I witnessed her expressing her remaining mental and physical abilities. Often I felt refreshed when I left the nursing home, as if I'd been on vacation. In a way, I had. My worries, deadlines, fears, and even physical pain had all been on hiatus for those hours, because I had been present and attentive during every moment with Mom.

Before becoming Mom's companion on the journey through Alzheimer's, I'd been practicing mindfulness meditation for over twenty-five years, and I had learned from Chödrön that "we don't sit in meditation to become good meditators. We sit in meditation so that we will be more awake in our lives."[41] While I sat quietly in meditation for twenty minutes every morning during those years I spent with Mom, many practical difficulties, intellectual challenges, and uncomfortable feelings about our situation did erupt during the silence. When this happened, my previous years of mindfulness practice served me well. By staying awake to everything, I was given an opportunity to recognize, accept, and process my feelings about the eruption, to carefully consider alternatives, and then freely choose to move forward toward communion and healing.

Caregivers who are just beginning to focus on being present in the moment will appreciate knowing in advance that courage (to face challenging, unpleasant, and ambivalent feelings and unwelcomed circumstances) and persistence are needed for us to be and stay fully present to what is happening in every moment. Persons with Alzheimer's do it naturally. Let them guide us.

The Gifts of Alzheimer's

Practices such as surrender, acceptance, and being present in the moment have their roots in ancient multifaith spirituality. Gratitude, another practice with spiritual roots, becomes especially significant in the context of Alzheimer's care because it encompasses the potential for healing brokenness and transcending loss and suffering. As we practice letting go, accepting what is, and being mindful, our abilities to glimpse and touch gratitude—even in the most difficult of circumstances—will become enhanced. Being aware of each and every one of Mom's accomplishments, no matter how small, seeing her smile when she recognized my arrival, and so many other hallowed little moments of every day in our life together made my soul sing in thanksgiving.

Benedictine and Zen monk Brother David Steindl-Rast offers a challenge to his students when he suggests that God is benevolent and gives only good gifts. With this theological position as his springboard, Steindl-Rast suggests that we consider being grateful for everything we're given in life—even if we consider it to be bad.[42] Persons with Alzheimer's and their loved ones may find this a particularly thorny theological position to consider, much less embrace. Alzheimer's a gift? Most of us—whether we have it or a loved one has it—would consider

Alzheimer's a curse. Jane Thibault and Richard Morgan write that even caregivers of deep faith will ask, "Why has God let this happen to us?" or "How can I go on believing in the goodness of God when I see Mom [Dad] suffering from a disease that destroys [her/his] memory and the person I know?"[43]

As I pondered these questions in the context of Alzheimer's, I reread the book of Job from the Hebrew Bible. Poor Job loses everything that he considers important in his external life: his family, his possessions, his wealth, and his health. According to ancient Hebrew theology, God punishes only those who have sinned. Through the lens of this theology, witnesses to Job's downfall and misery logically conclude that he must have sinned and that he therefore deserves his current situation as divine retribution.

Rabbi Harold Kushner, author of the insightful book *When Bad Things Happen to Good People*, consoled me during numerous times of loss and suffering throughout my life. With his analysis of the Book of Job, Kushner once again offered theological consolation as I confronted the realities of Alzheimer's disease. Rabbi Kushner notices that Job is sure of one thing, his own innocence. "Job, for his part, is unwilling to hold the world together theologically by admitting that he is a villain,"[44] and thereby deserving of the suffering he has received, presumably as a result of God's wrath. Job, who, according to Marcus Borg, is considered by many as a "voice of subversive and alternative wisdom,"[45] refuses to spare God's reputation. Kushner agrees: "He knows a lot of things intellectually, but he knows one thing more deeply. Job is absolutely sure that he is not a bad person."[46]

Translator and scholar Stephen Mitchell notes, that in his suffering, Job represents every man, every woman, "grieving for all of human misery."[47] In the early sections of Job's story, his despair increases because he doesn't realize or accept that wretched conditions and circumstances are part of our human destiny. For several years, my days were spent in a nursing home filled with persons with Alzheimer's who were collectively like Job. They too had lost almost everything of external importance: eyesight, hearing, mobility, limbs, speech, cognition, spouses, children, homes, pets, money and possessions, bladder and bowel control, the ability to feed themselves, the ability to chew and swallow, autonomy, and freedom. Their losses and misery, however, didn't exist solely because of their lives in a nursing home or because they had Alzheimer's. Elders and others I know who are healthy, independent, mentally sharp, active, and productive have experienced some of the same losses and pain that Job and the persons with Alzheimer's in the nursing home experienced. They have lost spouses, friends, children, homes, security, social position and respect, hearing, and teeth.

None of us is immune to loss, grief, suffering, and death. The longer we live, the more we will encounter, and witness in the lives of others. Longevity is currently identified as our greatest risk factor for getting Alzheimer's.

The writer of the book of Job has invited me to integrate this reality about loss and longevity into my beliefs about God and my witness of suffering and death as it relates to persons with Alzheimer's and their loved ones—none of whom deserve this disease, but all of whom must endure it. Accepting our inevitable diminishment as part of the human condition may, ironically, aid in alleviating the suffering connected with the diminishments of Alzheimer's. A Buddhist saying illustrates the wisdom beneath this acceptance: "If I break my leg, then I have pain. If I think there is a world where I should not have pain, then I suffer."

Mitchell's analysis of the book of Job helped me to see the intersection of loss, suffering, Alzheimer's, and God in a new way:

There is never an answer to the great question of life and death, unless it is my answer or yours. Because ultimately it isn't a question answered, but a person. Our whole being has to be answered. . . . When Job says, "I have heard of you with my ears; but now with my eyes have seen you," he is no longer a servant, who fears god and avoids evil. He has faced evil, has looked straight into its face and through it, into a vast wonder and love.[48]

Job's words describe another example of his alternative wisdom. Previously, he has heard about God only from what was written in the Hebrew scriptures. But with his own eyes, through his own being and presence, through his own agony, and at the lowest point in his life, Job has an extraordinary experience of the Divine. This experience changes his connection to God, Borg explains, from one of secondhand belief to one of firsthand relationship.[49]

Through their theological inquiries into the suffering of Job, both Kushner and Mitchell conclude that God is good. I found Kushner's words to be a guiding light on this subject: "[God] can still be on our side when bad things happen to us . . . we can turn to [God] for help." Our question, our prayer, and our petition will not be Job's question, 'God why are you doing this to me?' but rather, 'God see what is happening to me. Can You help me?' We will turn to God not to be judged or forgiven, not to be rewarded or punished, but to be strengthened and comforted."[50]

If caregivers can faithfully practice awareness and patience, if we can affirm that the Spirit of Life is present in all persons and working in different ways to manifest potential and call us toward goodness, and if we can accept the distress that we endure while trying to relieve the suffering of our loved ones, we may find our way *through* the anguish, as Job does—into vast wonder and love. After the intense misery that results from insisting he doesn't deserve loss and pain and demanding that things should be different, Job finally receives deep peace—by accepting reality.

If we can accept the perspectives about suffering and life offered by Steindl-Rast, Kushner, and Mitchell, we open ourselves to other possibilities. This opening calls forth another spiritual challenge. *If* there are good gifts in bad experiences, such as starving children, nuclear menace, natural disasters, the diminishment of aging, and the losses from Alzheimer's, Mitchell emphasizes, these gifts are buried somewhere under the devastating rubble of reality.[51] Once again, we are required to look, and to look hard. *Look* for strength. *Look* for comfort. *Look* for the choice between life and death.

Steindl-Rast, acknowledging—even for himself—the difficulty of looking for good gifts within hard experiences, further explains this invitation: "Gratefulness is the full response of the human heart to reality—as it is. Not to this reality or that reality." Anticipating our resistance to gratitude in the face of something that ought not to be there: outrageous words, actions, or experiences, and incurable diseases, for example, Steindl-Rast reassures us that he is not instructing us to be grateful for that which has outraged or distressed us. He is inviting us to be grateful in the face of these realities because, by acknowledging them, we are being given the opportunity to do something about them.[52]

I had been given the opportunity to make Mom's quality of life as good as it could be, to comfort her, and to protect her in small and large ways. These kinds of acts of love, according to Steindl-Rast, are expressions of "thanksgiving for the insights of love's vision."[53] My decision to care for Mom was born of my sense of belonging to her and her to me. Flowing out of this belonging, the service we caregivers offer to our loved ones is our expression of gratitude for being given the opportunity to serve. "On strong wings," Steindl-Rast writes, "love rises to every opportunity and shows itself grateful for it."[54]

My regular mindfulness practice increased the fruits of my intention to recognize and receive gifts and to feel gratitude in the midst of Mom's relentless decline. For me, one gift of having a loved one with Alzheimer's was the invitation to slow down. When I chose to walk slowly, matching Mom's pace, the words of Buddhist teacher Thich Nhat Hanh came to life: "In daily life there is so much to do and so little time. We feel pressured to run all the time. Just stop! Touch the ground of the present moment deeply, and you will touch real peace and joy."[55] I looked—really looked—at the flowers and the birds Mom so loved, examining their intricate details. Doing this heightened my desire and my ability to be present to life, and enlivened my enjoyment of every moment. I also chose to speak slowly and simply, increasing the opportunity for Mom to comprehend verbal communication. Consciously choosing not to complete her sentences with words I thought she might say, I waited patiently for her own words to emerge.[56] I listened to *her* and looked closely at *her*.

For both of us, every day was a new day of discovery. And every day, I was given opportunities to notice, accept, and love Mom, who she was, where she was. Every day brought opportunities to identify and meet her constantly changing needs. Embedded within these opportunities was the merging of love and gratefulness. Observing Mom's declining abilities and opening my heart to her brought me life's greatest gift, the experience of feeling and expressing unconditional love.

Being Mom's legal guardian manifested gifts born of a different kind of loving. The State of Iowa had empowered me to literally *be* Mom's voice. I spoke, not just on her behalf, but I spoke *as* her. As opportunities arose to help her by speaking up or taking action, I was most grateful for this gift of power. When she seemed sick, when I perceived her to be in danger, or when I concluded that her needs were being overlooked or neglected, I was not a helpless bystander, fretting and complaining to friends or wishing that things could be different. I could intervene to make things different. I had the power to seek hospice care for Mom, to change her doctor to someone who communicated well with cognitively impaired persons, to find out what kind of additional benefits were available to her (speech therapy, for example), to question the nursing home policies and procedures, to recommend interventions, to choose the aides who would work with Mom, to make dietary requests, and much more.

In one instance, when antibiotics no longer worked to cure Mom's recurring urinary tract infections, her doctor prescribed an herbal remedy. This was an unusual protocol for Mom's nursing home, and the nursing staff objected vehemently. If there was a chance this herb would relieve Mom's pain and discomfort, I didn't intend to allow the nursing home's objections to stand in the way.

Believing this remedy was in Mom's best interest and knowing that it would not harm her, I did something about it. It was hard and stressful for me to be a thorn in the side of the nursing home administration by taking a firm stand about this issue, but I found myself feeling grateful for the opportunity to push beyond my fears of upsetting people and do what was right for Mom. Through the Iowa Council on Aging, I located the nursing home ombudsman, who researched precedence and protocols for administering herbal prescriptions in Iowa. She then met with the nursing home administrator and nursing director and ensured that Mom's remedy would be administered as prescribed by her doctor.

After this episode was resolved, I felt as if I'd been through a war. The herb ultimately helped to relieve Mom's infections for a few months, so the battle felt rewarding. The stress and frustration I had endured, and even my subsequent battle fatigue, transformed into gifts. I felt grateful for the embodied reminder that I had worked relentlessly, and successfully, to relieve the suffering of a vulnerable and helpless being.

Our hardest experiences can be our best gifts because these experiences "make us grow the most," writes Steindl-Rast. [57] We don't, however, always appreciate the hard experiences the Universe brings to us. And no one, including Steindl-Rast, expects us to give thanks because the epidemic of Alzheimer's has touched our world, our loved ones, or our selves. He does encourage us, though, to focus our attention in reality, and from there, to try to find something—any tiny thing—for which we can sincerely give thanks.

Embarking on a quest to make meaning from the challenges in our lives—including those inherent in Alzheimer's—is one way to deepen our gratitude for all that is. More often, though, as T. S. Eliot writes, "we have the experience but miss the meaning." [58] Richard Rohr reminds us that medical advances have given us more years but adds that we don't have good models for how to live these additional years, which include ever-expanding health challenges and diminishments, in ways that will bring deeper meaning to our lives. [59]

Regarding Alzheimer's care, I agree. We don't have models for finding deeper meaning. In 1973, my smart, feisty, independent mother was diagnosed with breast cancer. She survived long enough to manifest Alzheimer's disease thirty-five years later. Mom's story of surviving into Alzheimer's is similar for millions of elders. What is the purpose of this survival? Where is the deeper meaning?

"In some ways suffering ceases to be suffering at the moment it finds a meaning," writes concentration camp survivor, Viktor Frankl." [60] Steindl-Rast defines meaning through metaphor, "the light in which we see things." [61] As we seek the ability to bear our circumstances through deeper meaning in life and to find reasons to be grateful, our hearts naturally thirst for this light. It's important to keep in mind that our loved ones with Alzheimer's have not abandoned this inherently human quest. Their hearts also thirst for the light of meaning that is as life-giving to humans as sunlight. Just as they need us to walk with them out into the sunlight, persons with Alzheimer's also need us to walk with them into the light of meaning. Their loss of autonomy makes relationship an essential element in their ongoing quest.

Persons with Alzheimer's express their appreciation for our attention and care in ways we will need to endeavor to interpret. For years, I witnessed nursing aides tenderly caring for my mother and many others with Alzheimer's—a mostly verbally silent population—without expecting or needing a word of thanks. They had learned to feel appreciated by knowing the meaningfulness of their work and the the gratefulness that beamed forth from a smile, or a nod, or a touch from their residents.

If persons with Alzheimer's could talk, I believe most would graciously express gratitude for the care and attention they are receiving in the midst of an outrageous, unconquerable experience of diminishment. I make this prediction based on my own observations. History, however, also reveals to us that suffering, vulnerable people are grateful for any kindnesses, and that they can have a life-changing impact on others. In 1889, writer Robert Louis Stevenson visited a hospital in Hawaii specifically for patients suffering with Hansen's disease, more commonly known as leprosy. Six years earlier, Mother Marianne Cope, a Franciscan nun from New York, was asked to establish this hospital, which became known as the Bishop Home. Isolated from the rest of society by law, disfigured by disease, persons with leprosy had long been society's outcasts. In caring for this population, Mother Marianne insisted on cleanliness, music, and beauty—to help put a little more sunshine into their dreary lives.[62] I can't help but compare them to the scores of persons with cognitive decline now considered outcasts by society.

After visiting Bishop Home, Stevenson wrote this poem affirming Mother Marianne's work.

To see the infinite pity of this place,
The mangled limb, the devastated face
The innocent sufferers smiling at the nod,
A fool were tempted to deny his God.

He sees and shrinks, but if he look again,
Lo, beauty springing from the breast of pain.
He honors the sisters on those painful shores,
And even a fool is silent and adores.[63]

Stevenson's words express his awareness of gratefulness as Steindl-Rast defines it, "full aliveness" held together by the heartbeat of this present moment.[64] He memorializes his own gratefulness for the sisters' ministry and his recognition of the gratefulness of the "innocent sufferers" who smile at the slightest acknowledgment of their existence. In addition, Stevenson shares the meaning he harvested from "looking again," a deepening of his relationship with the Holy.

As I heard stories of illness and pain from persons with Alzheimer's and their caregivers, and witnessed their losses and suffering, I also witnessed acceptance, joy, and gratefulness in spite of it all. In my search to understand how people of faith could accept and transcend the losses of aging and Alzheimer's disease, I arrived at the intersection of process theology and liberation theology. According to theologian C. Robert Mesle, process theology teaches that the life-giving energy of the Universe works in relational ways to help guide us to freedom and healing.[65] Liberation theology interprets the teachings of Jesus in terms of the essential need to liberate the poor and the suffering from unjust economic, political, or social conditions. As I considered the innocent sufferers I encountered through this inquiry—Job, the persons with leprosy at the Bishop Home, and the persons with Alzheimer's in Mom's nursing home—and as I searched for meaning, the combined perspectives of process theology and liberation theology brought me comfort and inspired me. Stevenson was inspired to silent adoration by his witness of "beauty springing from the breast of pain." Similarly, I was inspired as I encountered the undeserved pain of persons with Alzheimer's and their caregivers. Noticing the healing relationship between the Spirit of Life and humanity strengthened my belief in the ultimate holiness in all of life.[66]

Through my empathic, relational witness of Mom's decline, I felt called to leave my busy life in Boston and to walk slowly with her on the last steps on her journey "home." Answering yes to this call was an acknowledgment of my understanding of Mesle's idea that "God's primary avenue to liberation [of the suffering] is through responsive human hearts."[67] My yes to caring for Mom became the greatest honor and the greatest gift of my life.

The millions of other caregivers who are offering love and care to persons with Alzheimer's have also been called to serve through relational witness and awareness. Without question, this call is difficult to receive, and even more, difficult to wholeheartedly accept; it is perhaps the hardest experience of our lives so far. If, however, we consider the possibility that there are gifts in the midst of our difficulties, if we look consciously at our frustrations, sadness, burdens, and sacrifices, we will notice opportunities for enhancing our abilities to observe and accept what is, to be present, and to feel grateful. All of this encompasses the heartbeat of the spiritual journey. In these places of loss and suffering—places where we don't expect to find anything of value or of beauty—springs the possibility that we will open ourselves to meeting our loved ones with Alzheimer's in mutuality, to receiving grace, and to experiencing gratefulness.

Alzheimer's disease is giving us countless invitations to do something and to receive the gift of knowing that we can make a difference. We can

- lobby Congress for more funding for research
- work to find cause and cure by participating in fundraisers such as the Walk to End Alzheimer's
- visit persons with Alzheimer's at care centers and nursing homes or through hospice organizations
- urge care centers, nursing homes, and home-care providers to become more informed about and trained to deliver the specialized care needed for persons with Alzheimer's
- insist that our loved ones and others with Alzheimer's be treated with understanding, kindness, and dignity
- establish more social awareness and understanding so persons with Alzheimer's can become more actively engaged in their communities
- find ways to transform our personal pain and loss into meaningful, healing experiences for our selves, our loved ones, and others who are touched by this disease

Seeking and finding opportunities to make a healing difference in our own lives or the lives of others—is the most effective antidote to feeling helpless. Using what we learn through our difficult experiences to enlighten, encourage, and assist others is the most effective prescription for transforming heartbreak into gratitude.

Believing in Relationship

Choose Love. Without it, this beautiful Love,
Life is nothing but a burden.

—Rumi

The path of Alzheimer's is so highly unpredictable. As my caregiving companions (including families, medical professionals, and scientists) and I walked this path with persons with the disease, we lived the questions the world is asking about the meaning and purpose of Alzheimer's. We were often challenged by what we encountered along the way. More often, we were surprised. There is no doubt that the path we walked along with persons with Alzheimer's was not always clear. Our role in the lives of our loved ones, however, was always clear. Our role was to love them every step of the way.

One of the great unknowns on this journey through Alzheimer's is how long a person will live with this disease. Although it's designated as a terminal illness because there is no cure, some consider Alzheimer's to be a disability since afflicted persons can live with declining abilities for four to twenty years.[1] Rather than preparing for an imminent death, seemingly endless adapting is required.

This long journey home for persons who have Alzheimer's will eventually lead to a fork in the road. One path leads them into silence, isolation, and loneliness. The other path, relationship, leads them to a life rich with communication, connection, meaning, and love. Because of the dependent nature of Alzheimer's, especially during the advanced stages, family caregivers and caring professionals will determine which path those afflicted will travel.

My eighty-two-year-old friend Constance knows that Alzheimer's afflicts 50 percent of people over eighty-five. She is in remarkably good health; however, she still fears that she will get this disease. Constance is not alone. The *New York Times* reports that Americans are more afraid of Alzheimer's than of dying.[2] Constance expressed her fear to a friend, who consoled her and calmed her fears by saying, "Well, if there is someone who understands the disease to love you and take really good care of you, maybe it wouldn't be so bad."

Increasing our understanding and our loving will best qualify us to be effective caregivers for and companions to persons with Alzheimer's on their journeys home. This effort, however, will also enhance our own journeys. Our own healing begins in true encounter with others.

Moving more deeply into the world of meaningful relationships . . .

The Most Important Memories

At the door to the memory unit in one care facility I toured, I was greeted by a sign bearing the prophetic words of poet Maya Angelou: "People will forget what you said, people will forget what you did, but people will never forget how you made them feel."

Angelou's words reminded me of an important reality about being human: our emotions matter. They inform our decisions. They guide our reactions. They express our deep truths. Unfortunately, our rational, intellectual, technological, fast-paced world tends to ignore this reality, even for the healthiest of us. The emotions of those who are limited in their abilities to actually identify and communicate their feelings in traditionally expected ways are even more unacknowledged. Aware and enlightened Alzheimer's caregivers have known for quite a long time, however, that Angelou's recognition is true for *all* people, even for cognitively impaired people.

At a dementia care conference, I was introduced to the poem "Heart Memories," written by Louise Eder in 1984. Although I couldn't find out if Louise is/was a person with Alzheimer's, a family carepartner, or a professional caregiver, her poem reveals

her understanding of the retention and importance of emotions
in persons with Alzheimer's.

I remember you with my heart
My mind won't say your name
I can't recall where or if I knew you
Who you were or who I was.

Maybe I grew up with you or
Maybe we worked together
Or did we bowl together yesterday?
There's something wrong with my
Memory but I do know you—and I
Do love you.

I know I knew you
I know how you make me feel
I remember the feelings we had together
My heart remembers
It cries out in loneliness for you
For the feelings you give me now.

Today I'm happy that you have come
When you leave
My mind will not remember that
You were here
But my heart remembers
Remembers the feeling of friendship
And love returned
Remembers
That I am less lonely and happier
Today because of the feeling
Because you have come

Please don't forget me
And please don't stay away
Because of the way my mind acts.
I can still feel you
I can still remember you with my heart
And a heart memory is maybe
The most important memory of all.[3]

As the publication date of *Heart Memories* indicates, some caregivers have long known that it remains possible to connect deeply and maintain meaningful relationships with persons experiencing the brain alterations associated with Alzheimer's and dementia. These caregivers have recognized and appreciated the existence and the power of emotions, emotional expression, and emotional memory in persons with Alzheimer's. For more than twenty years, Dr. Paul Raia has provided care and support to persons with Alzheimer's and their families through his work with the Alzheimer's Association in Massachusetts. Before moving to Iowa, I had the great honor of meeting with Raia, a true innovator in the discipline of Alzheimer's care. Two decades ago, he started the first support groups for persons with early-stage dementia and for young children with grandparents or parents with Alzheimer's or a related dementia. From the onset of his work with Alzheimer's, Dr. Raia focused his attention on the cognitively impaired persons' emotions and their remaining capacities.

Through his commitment to observing the reality of Alzheimer's through "the collective experience of caregivers," Raia recognized that

the capacity to feel and exhibit emotions persists among people with Alzheimer's disease far into the disease process. What is lost is the insight into what might have triggered a particular emotion or how to control it. The

ability to feel emotions, then, may be our best inroad to
the mind of the person with Alzheimer's disease.[4]

Raia's understanding of the enduring, and even heightened, life of the emotions in persons with Alzheimer's disease
echoes my improvisation teachers' guidance away from saying
no. He explains that when we say no, our muscles automatically
tense and the tone of our voice changes, which persons with
Alzheimer's will notice.[5]

Writer Colleen Carroll Campbell, another daughter of a
person with Alzheimer's, shared her observations of this dynamic:
"Dad's memory may have been ravaged in those last years, but
his emotional acuity was keener than ever. Like an infant reacting to the stresses in his surroundings, Dad's mood was might-
ily affected by the tone of voice and gentleness or harshness
of another's touch."[6] With their heightened sensitivity to body
language and voice cues, persons with Alzheimer's will instinctively interpret expressions of no as controlling or demeaning,
and they will react. Raia reminds us that, because of their limited ability to communicate verbally, "the situation becomes
highly emotional."[7] "No," as well as other emotionally charged
words uttered without thought and actions taken without consideration, can deflate or incite persons with Alzheimer's.

In relationship with persons who are very emotionally sensitive, our abilities to feel and name our own emotions will
increase our empathy and enhance our understanding of others and our effectiveness as caregivers. At a Healing Moments
workshop, neuroscientist and author Lisa Genova participated in
an exercise in which the leader said no to her about something
important. Lisa felt and named her emotions and reactions:

> Here is the exercise I remember most. I was asked to say
> a simple statement, something I believe to be true. I said,
> smiling, "I have the most beautiful six-month old boy."

The instructor, looking me straight in the eye and without smiling, said, "You do not have a six-month old baby. Your kids are all grown. You don't know what you're talking about."

My turn came around again.

"It's a glorious, sunny day outside."

"No, it's not. It's dark and cloudy, and it's going to rain."

Here's what I noticed. Even though I knew this was just an exercise: I didn't want to talk with this woman. I didn't like being told I was wrong, I didn't like the look on her face, and I didn't like her tone of voice. In fact, I felt my emotions stirred by the interaction, like I was readying to argue or fight.[8]

Being aware of our own emotional reactions can help us understand why persons with Alzheimer's react as they do. Statements they make are as true for them as having a beautiful baby boy was true for Lisa. This awareness can be a catalyst for caregivers to change the ways we speak to and interact with persons with Alzheimer's. By doing so, we may ease their suffering and perhaps even manage behaviors previously managed with medication.

To Raia's collective experience of caregivers, I add my own observations of my mother's capability to feel and communicate her emotions. During my years in Iowa, it was my practice to spend time with Mom every day, often in the morning and through her lunchtime. Alternately, I was with her for dinner, followed by an evening walk or an activity. I would usually stay until bath time or bedtime. Sometimes, especially if she was not feeling well, I was with her for both lunch and dinner. Clearly, she had become accustomed to seeing and being with me every day.

On a few occasions, I needed to return to Massachusetts for professional reasons. Intentionally, my trips were short, never more than four days. During my first trip, the nurses charted Mom's emotional pattern. They reported that she was fine the first day. By the second evening, she seemed withdrawn. The next morning, she didn't want to eat. She was lethargic and slept more than usual. No amount of coaxing, cajoling, or entertaining would convince her to smile.

When I returned, I went directly from the airport to the nursing home. It was dinnertime, and Mom was already sitting at her place at the table, which faced the door to the dining room. Always attentive to movement around her, Mom noticed me as soon as I walked in. I stopped, and our eyes met. It took a few seconds for recognition to register, but suddenly her whole face—her entire being—registered joy. She started speaking excitedly in her own language of sounds. She couldn't seem to stop chattering on and on about my arrival. She hugged me tightly, then held my hands and wouldn't let go. An aide had to feed her because neither Mom nor I had a free hand. In my entire life, I have never felt such acclaim. The staff was amazed by this display of emotion, and Mom's joy permeated the entire floor. Everyone seemed filled with happiness that night.

At first, I was sad and disappointed in myself because I interpreted Mom's distress and withdrawal while I was away as my failure to care for her well. I felt I shouldn't have left her. But my absence for four days wasn't exactly the cause of Mom's distress. She missed me, and missing me was a normal reaction for the situation. She was communicating her feelings in the only way she could, sadness manifested as withdrawal. The ultimate cause of Mom's distress was her decline from Alzheimer's and her lost capacities as they intersected with my absence.

Perhaps Mom was also feeling afraid that I wouldn't return. Raia explains, "Patients with Alzheimer's disease experience fear throughout their disease course. As they decline and lose capacities, part of what is also lost is the ability to articulate their fears and cope with them. Essentially, what is lost is the person's ability to self-soothe if fears become overwhelming."[9] Without the ability to comfort herself, Mom was at the mercy of all sorts of unrealistic fears.

During later trips that kept me away for several days, I arranged for hospice volunteers, nurses, or the reflexologist to spend time with Mom each day. I specifically asked them to do some of the activities with Mom that I did: brush her hair, massage her hands, walk with her outside, and take her to Mass and exercise class. Because she could not soothe herself, I asked them to reassure her that I was coming back very soon, and that I missed her too. This external soothing seemed to help stabilize her emotional state while I was away.

Colleen Carroll Campbell's father lived with Alzheimer's for fifteen years. She shares some of her family's struggle: "One of the hardest things about those years—especially for my mother, his faithful exhausted caregiver—was hearing well-intentioned people dismiss the need for her solicitous care or their own failure to visit him by saying that 'he doesn't remember anyway.'"[10] Sometimes it became necessary for me to defend myself against people with these opinions, including some members of my own family, who denied my mother's need for the care and attention I was giving to her. They were convinced that my daily presence in Mom's life was unnecessary because she didn't remember anyway. Having people question and criticize my good care of Mom was demoralizing and disempowering. In response, however, I could only assume that they didn't understand (or were afraid to understand) what it meant for a person to be completely vulnerable, completely helpless, and on their own in a nursing home, completely at the mercy of strangers. I also assumed that they didn't realize how important it is for vulnerable persons with Alzheimer's disease to have consistent, loving companionship.

Recently, Robert, a psychologist from Wisconsin, added his curiosity about the emotions of persons with Alzheimer's to the collective caregiver experience. At the time, his mother, Martha, was eighty-three years old and had moderately severe Alzheimer's disease. She lived in a care facility in a small town in southwestern Wisconsin, and Robert faithfully visited her every Thursday afternoon. There were times when Robert wondered whether his time visiting his mother was well spent. Did his visits actually make any difference to her? By the day after his visit—according to staff reports and his own assessment based on phone interactions with his mother—Martha would have cognitively forgotten whether her son had come or not. She seemed to have no memory of his visits.

One Thursday, Robert, swamped with work assignments, decided to skip his weekly visit. The next day, the charge nurse called him to report that Martha was in an unusually foul mood. She was agitated and seemed quite unhappy. They weren't sure why; nothing was different.

Robert wondered if Martha had missed his visit, even though she was cognitively incapable of remembering whether or not he had come at his usual time—or that he had come at all. Robert took this caregiver experience with him to a professional conference. To the good fortune of persons with Alzheimer's disease all around the world, he expressed his wonder to someone who listened with his heart: Daniel Tranel, professor of neurology and psychology, and director of the Neuroscience Graduate Program at the University of Iowa.[11]

Generally, scientists aren't all that interested in anecdotal evidence like Robert's story. After all, the world of science has passed over the anecdotal information expressed in *Heart Memories,* published almost thirty years ago, and Raia's writing about the "collective experience of caregivers" observing emotions in persons with Alzheimer's, published more than a decade ago. But Robert and Martha's story peaked Tranel's interest. The outcome will change the course of treatment for persons with Alzheimer's worldwide. It will improve their lives as well as the lives of their family members and care providers.

A scientific study published in 2010 by Iowa research-ers Justin Feinstein, Melissa Duff, and Daniel Tranel "provides direct evidence that a feeling of emotion can endure beyond the conscious recollection for the events that initially triggered the emotion."[12] These insightful researchers understand the meaning of their findings. They state, "The results of this study have direct implications for how society treats individuals with memory disorders (such as persons with Alzheimer's disease), since events that have long been forgotten could continue to induce suffering or well being." For example, visits or telephone calls from family members to persons with Alzheimer's could positively influence their affective states. These positive feel-ings could linger even if the visits or phone calls are forgotten. On the other hand, neglect from family members and routine neglect and insensitive treatment by staff at nursing homes may leave cognitively impaired persons feeling sad, frustrated, angry, and lonely, even though they can't remember why. The study results show that these upsetting feelings tend to linger longer than the happier feelings.[13]

Many, including some who work directly with persons with Alzheimer's, desperately need to be informed about this research. At a dementia care conference, I met one nursing aide working in a mid-western nursing home who spoke for many, I'm afraid, when she said of her residents with Alzheimer's, "It doesn't matter how we treat them. They don't know the dif-ference anyway." I gasp at this inhumane, uninformed attitude. Infants know the difference. Animals know the difference. Even plants respond to encouraging words and a gentle touch!

In a summary of their findings, the Iowa researchers offer this profound conclusion: "As the number of individuals suf-fering from Alzheimer's disease, and other forms of dementia, reaches epidemic proportions, it will be imperative for society to follow a scientifically informed standard of care for patients with memory impairments."[14] They have statistically proven that the level of well-being or suffering for persons with Alzheimer's could continue long after they have cognitively forgotten how others interacted with them.

Now, the anecdotes we caregivers notice and share, such as the following story, will be credited with validity as well as fused with poignancy:

Each summer at Mom's nursing home, the family of one of the residents brought Shetland ponies that pulled buggies with fringes on top. They took residents, family members, and staff for rides. While Mom and I rode in the buggy, she could not take her eyes, which were dancing with delight, off that pony. After our ride, she petted the pony and fed him a carrot. I noticed that Mom's neighbor Etty, an avid animal lover, was obviously cheered to the core of her being by the ponies. Her shining eyes and big smile radiated joy. About fifteen minutes later, I saw Etty upstairs near her room. She was smiling, laughing, and bouncy. But when I exclaimed, "You really enjoyed those ponies, didn't you!" Etty's expression became completely puzzled. She stopped bouncing and smiling and seemed disturbed.

She asked, "What? What are you talking about?"

I felt terrible about interrupting her cheerful pony mood, so I patted her arm, hugged her, and said, "I'm so happy to see you, Etty."

Then I smiled and laughed. She smiled and laughed, and the pony cheer seemed to resurface as she bounced off down the hallway.

I was shocked by how quickly Etty had cognitively forgotten the pony experience, which had so delighted her. It had just been minutes. I tried to imagine what it would be like to not remember something that happened moments ago, but of course I couldn't really grasp it. Etty's reaction to my question told me that her cognitive decline was progressing. Her short-term cognitive memory could not reach back even minutes, but her emotional memory lingered. This momentary interaction heightened my awareness and alerted me that I needed to adjust my communication with Etty according to her abilities to help her maintain a positive emotional state. This experience also reminded me of the importance of paying attention to inevitable changes in cognition.

Numerous researchers have studied the effects of emotion on cognitive memory, but until Dr. Tranel's curiosity was sparked by Robert and Martha's story, scientists knew very little about how memory affects emotion. Initially, the Iowa study considered this intriguing question: Is the "sustained experience of an emotion dependent upon, versus independent of, intact declarative memory for the events that initially caused the emotion?"[15]

On behalf of the collective caregiver experience, I can confidently answer no to this question. Sustained emotions in persons with Alzheimer's are not dependent on being able to cognitively remember or verbally express what stimulated that emotion. Unfortunately, our society is not programmed to pay attention to stories of individual experiences, even when they've been collected. Although physicians and psychologists have reported for years on the critical nature of individualized phenomenology (what we can observe) as it relates to Alzheimer's care, our society is programmed to pay attention only to statistical data. Therefore, these scientists in Iowa have done a great service to persons with memory loss caused by damage to the hippocampus, the part of the brain responsible for forming, organizing, and storing memories.[16] They have provided data. For many years, Raia has been telling society that we needed this data: "Developing a better understanding of the psychology of dementia—how a person thinks, feels, communicates, compensates, and responds to change, to emotion, to love—may bring some of the biggest breakthroughs in treatment."[17]

Here the scientific breakthrough has arrived! Feeling, however, that their observations and insights have been overlooked, some family caregivers and professionals in the field reacted with frustration to the attention now being given to the data. "We don't need a study to tell us what we already know, what we have known all along!" It's true—many caregivers don't need this evidence. Those who have chosen to become intimately involved with persons with Alzheimer's know that the damage to their brains has not interfered with their heart memories. The difference between validation by data and validation by story regarding the emotional memory of persons with Alzheimer's reminds me of Joseph Campbell's comment said during "The Power of Myth" interviews. PBS commentator Bill Moyers asked Campbell if he had faith in God. He replied, "I don't need faith. I have experience."[18]

The caregiver collective has experience. And our experience has made us believers. The rest of the world, however, does *not* have this experience. And, in the absence of experience, doubt flourishes. Doctors Feinstein, Duff, and Tranel are not telling caregivers what we already know. They are confirming what we know. In addition, they are telling the rest of the world what it doesn't know, what it needs to know, what it *must* know.

This scientific data has the power to demand a major reformation in the field of Alzheimer's caregiving. For example, the study results suggest that behavioral problems exhibited by persons with Alzheimer's could stem from sadness or anxiety that they cannot explain.[19] The current trend of care, which tends to medicate behavioral issues (usually to the detriment, and sometimes resultant death,[20] of the person with Alzheimer's), *must* change. And it will change—because now, scientific data "provides clear evidence showing that the reasons for treating [persons with Alzheimer's and dementia-type memory loss] with respect and dignity go beyond simple human morals."[21]

It seems wrong to some dedicated caregivers that data, more so than experience of the individual, should dictate a standard of appropriate care. And so the caregivers cry out, "Why do we need scientists to tell us that persons with Alzheimer's should be morally considered and treated with respect and dignity?" My voice was part of this cry when I first read the Iowa study. After living with this question, however, I eventually found an answer: Because now we caregivers have validation of our experiential knowing that the world understands and accepts. Essentially, this study on emotional memory has given the individual caregiver experience clout. The next time a nonbeliever (a family member, a friend, or even an uninformed, untrained professional) questions our dedication to caring for our loved ones with dignity and our commitment to relating to them as valuable members of our lives and our world, we can confidently, powerfully say, "Research has shown . . ."

The Iowa researchers have given caregivers even more than data and clout, however. By showing us that one story told to one person can make a world of difference to millions, the Iowa researchers have given us hope.

Time Enough

I n the Iowa town that I once again call home, Alzheimer's caregivers gather every year in the rose garden at the arboretum. In this place of peacefulness and breathtaking beauty, we gather to honor our loved ones who are living with Alzheimer's and to remember those who have been liberated by death from the disease they have endured for so long. Year after year, we gather to participate in a ritual of release. As each loved one's name is called, a chime rings and the resonant sound unites with the wind. We watch in awe, reverence, and delight as carepartners release Monarch butterflies, freeing them to continue their natural process of life and death.

During the first flight of their life journeys, our butterflies dazzle us with their beauty. But their time for dazzling will be brief. They live very short lives—two to six weeks. This fact of nature, of each ending life, brings us sadness. The Indian poet Rabindrinath Tagore consoles us as we contemplate this truth:

The butterfly counts not months but moments,
and has time enough.[22]

"Time enough for what?" I found myself asking. The answer was surprising.

During their short lives, Monarchs have time enough to lay their eggs. Thus, they participate in creating the next migrating generation, which will miraculously travel from our rose garden in Iowa to the fir trees their ancestors inhabited last winter in Mexico. The migrating generation of Monarchs won't just travel to the same country, the same town, or even the same neighborhood of their ancestors. Relying solely on the guidance of their natural instincts and the instincts of their companions, they will travel to the exact same trees.

The migrating generation will need time enough to make their long flight home, and to then lay their eggs. So, unlike our butterflies—whose lives are fleeting—the migrating Monarchs live eight months or more.

Each generation of Monarchs has time enough to fulfill its purpose.

"Time is the most valuable thing we have, because it is the most irrevocable," wrote Dietrich Bonhoeffer from a Nazi prison cell during World War II.[23] Like someone who has received the diagnosis of a terminal illness, Bonhoeffer *knew* that his days on earth were limited. His precarious state of imprisonment heightened his awareness about the preciousness of each passing moment and the importance of each word he wrote or spoke.

Building on Bonhoeffer's thought, Jewish scholar and mystic Abraham Joshua Heschel believes that "time is the heart of existence." When I was first introduced to Heschel's teachings about time, I felt that he had given me a map for travelling through life in a different way. Like many, I thought that sacred images or sacred places, such as art or churches or nature, were the doorways to experiencing mystery. With Heschel's encouragement, I began to consider the nature of *time* in my quest for God and meaning in life. "The higher goal of spiritual living," writes Heschel, "is to face sacred moments.... What is retained in the soul is the moment of insight rather than the place where the act took place." He encouraged me to build a "sanctuary in time…where the goal is not to have but to be, not to own but to give, not to control but to share, not to subdue, but to be in accord."[24] Inspired by this possibility, I was able to create such a sanctuary for Mom and me in the sacred time we had left together.

It's now abundantly clear to me that our choices regarding the gift of time we have been given do matter. Our loved ones with Alzheimer's may live for twenty years with this disease. If we can discover ways to make these additional years of life meaningful for them, and for us, then the longevity medical science gives us can be a blessing. This search for meaning remains a mysterious, holy quest whose answer we, and our loved ones, must live into—over time.

The process of diminishment from Alzheimer's intersects with the distinct life journey of each person with the disease as well as the journeys of their family members. Accordingly, the Alzheimer's experience is uniquely manifested.

The purpose of the journey and the value of the time that it gave to my caregiver companions and me varied, and what we each were able to give and to receive in our time enough sometimes surprised even us.

Writer Sherri Edwards shares with us that the "most meaningful present" her mother gave her was "the gift of walking with her on the path of a progressive illness," in this case vascular dementia. Although "shocked to admit this," Edwards was able to move beyond the "unbearable sadness at the loss of the mother [she] knew," to surmount her "struggle under the weight of increasing responsibilities," and to manage the despair and guilt she felt over neglecting the rest of her life. Having navigated her way through these challenging feelings, Edwards was able to recognize the blessings she received along the way.

Edwards and her mother have found purpose and value in their time enough. Even with dementia, her mother continues to be "a teacher, a counselor, a friend," who is "incredibly" still giving gifts. The first "gift" Sherri mentions receiving on this journey through dementia with her mother is the gift of *time*. "Many friends have lost parents years ago. Yet here is my mother, who has survived several serious illnesses plus dementia.... I am growing older with my mother right here, and I am grateful." Edwards also feels grateful for her mom's "warm and sincere hugs" and the way her mom's face light up whenever she enters the room. She is grateful for the opportunity to be a role model of caring and family loyalty for her children. She is grateful to have learned the lesson that "the little moments," like buttoning her mother's coat, count, and that blessings can be found in a life circumstance that "no one would ever wish for."[25]

As Edwards points out, our loved ones with Alzheimer's are still with us. Their very presence in our lives indicates that they have survived the many challenges of the twentieth century—medical and otherwise. As I contemplate the lives of our loved ones with Alzheimer's, I pause and recognize the contributions they have made—and continue to make—to our lives. Many of these diminishing persons, now eighty, ninety, or one hundred years old, courageously embarked as pioneers across oceans, prairies and deserts. Many have bravely shown us how to live through wars, holocausts, and depressions. And now, once again pioneers, many are showing us how to live with Alzheimer's disease. They are lighting the way for us as we travel through this mysterious and treacherous terrain.

Author Stephen Post, an important teacher and guide for me, begins his book *The Moral Challenge of Alzheimer's Disease* with these words: "Seldom does human experience require more courage than in living with the diagnosis and the gradual decline of irreversible progressive dementia." Post then asks,

"How can affected individuals and their caregivers maintain 'the courage to be' before the foreboding specter of dementia?"[26]

Fortunately, many children of persons with Alzheimer's have embraced their loved ones and the disease with a spirit born of love, vision, and healing. Many of these visionary daughters and sons (and spouses, relatives, and friends) are coming forward to share their witness of the transforming power of this disease. By doing so, they recognize, reveal, and model the importance of expressing our authentic selves, even when authenticity includes decline from Alzheimer's.

Conventional wisdom, unfortunately, still concludes that Alzheimer's steals personhood along with our opportunities to heal, reconcile, develop, or deepen our relationships with the persons who have this disease. However, we, the children of persons with Alzheimer's, have the clarity, confidence, and courage to share our alternative wisdom. We are revealing the gifts we have noticed and received. We are expressing awe and gratitude for the ways our encounters with Alzheimer's have transformed our lives. We are guiding society into the mystery of meaning and value. And we are revealing how our time enough has deepened our relationships with our loved ones and changed our lives forever.

Time Enough for Meeting

For more than fourteen years, Coleen was the primary caregiver for her mother, Ilene. Based on her experiences and observations, Coleen strongly disagrees with those who contend that people with Alzheimer's have forgotten who they are or who we are. Fearing that not enough members of our society have invested the time needed to meet people with Alzheimer's as they are and learn the skills needed to maintain relationships with them, she is concerned for their welfare. Knowing from the beginning that her understanding of this disease would be critical for her mother's well-being, Coleen sought out information. She also attempted to educate her brothers, who mostly avoided the subject. Instead of being angry with her brothers, Coleen chose to let them go, and they chose to let her "handle it." In the end, Coleen felt happy, satisfied, and content with her choices.

There were times earlier in Coleen's life when Ilene had guided and comforted her throughout challenging experiences—a painful ending to a serious relationship and the births of her babies, for example. Even while Ilene had Alzheimer's, Coleen continued to see her mother as her guide and comforter. There is a hereditary component for early-onset Alzheimer's, the type Ilene had. "Sometimes," Coleen said, "I looked at Mom, and I saw my future."

She saw her mother courageously and gracefully blazing the trail for her. This kind of terrifying awareness, which often sends adult children into avoidance, didn't cause Coleen to turn away from her mother's decline. Instead, she turned toward her mother, growing closer and nurturing their mother-daughter relationship, which transformed into a woman-to-woman connection.

Coleen believes that her fourteen-year journey with her mother through Alzheimer's disease gave her time enough to establish clear priorities in her life. Alzheimer's disease reminded Coleen of her own mortality and spurred her to complete her bachelor's degree in business so she can be satisfied with the contribution she is making to the world.[27] This long journey also gave Coleen time enough to learn more about herself. In many ways, Coleen's intimate meeting with her mother through Alzheimer's brought out the best in her, introducing her to an inner strength she didn't know she had. "I'm not that strong," she said. "But when it came to Mom, I just had to be strong. She needed help to have a good quality of life. Not just from anybody—she needed help from me."

Coleen and Ilene's years together on the Alzheimer's journey also gave them time enough for their connection to deepen into a relationship that Coleen considered "very holy." As the disease progressed and their relationship grew more intimate, Coleen, literally "became one" with her mother:

> I was her eyes, her ears, her voice. Because I had to 'be' her, our bond became unbreakable, and I truly felt as if I was accomplishing something very important. Although Mom couldn't speak, I knew that she was communicating with her eyes, and this drew me closer to her. No one at the nursing home could hear her or speak for her. She needed me to read her communications through her eyes and to communicate with words on her behalf. I felt strongly about being her caregiver, and it is something I will always be proud of—working on behalf of one of God's children who could not help herself.

There are family members who are "visitors" in nursing homes. With coaxing from Coleen, even her brothers eventually became visitors—and visitors are a good thing. According to an African proverb, "Visitors' footfalls are like medicine; they heal the sick." Coleen, however, was much more than a visitor. She was an active, assertive carepartner for her mother. Indeed, the hands-on care that Coleen gave Ilene—making sure the nursing home aides were respectful of her body, washing her up after toileting, walking with her, holding her memories, feeding her, and spending all night with her in the hospital so she wouldn't wake up and be alone and afraid—was holy work. Once when Ilene fell and was taken to the hospital, Coleen left work and rushed to her bedside in the emergency room. She instinctively knew that her mother would be confused and frightened. "*My* touch is what Mom needed," she says. "She needed *me* there to hold her hand." Coleen also knew from experience that most medical professionals require some clear direction when attending to a person with dementia who can't speak. And Coleen was there, without fail, to provide that direction.

At Ilene's deathbed, Coleen wept. After this long, deeply intimate journey together, Coleen was bereft because she couldn't figure out how to continue walking with her mom as she left this world. Their bond was that strong, that profound.

Throughout the many years that Coleen was a regular carepartner for Ilene at the nursing home, she continued to recognize the presence of God beaming through her mom's eyes and radiating through the warm hands of the other residents with Alzheimer's. Just as this presence remains recognizable to us, it's possible that the presence of God in our eyes and our hands remains recognizable to them as well.

Time Enough for Discovery

If we accept Brother David Steindl-Rast's definition of God as surprise,[28] then Mary Anne encountered God numerous times throughout her mother's diminishment from dementia. After Ione suffered her first seizure in 1997, the diagnosis of Alzheimer's was mentioned for the first time. Mary Anne remembers being filled with despair as she considered the possibility that her mother would lose her memory. After years of witnessing Ione's gradual decline, however, Mary Anne was surprised to discover that her fear of having a mother with dementia had been more painful than the reality: "It could have been so much worse. I know Mom had frustrations, but she didn't have pain. Now that I've been through it, I realize it was probably worse for us experiencing Mom's losses than it actually was for her.[29] She didn't seem to know, and she didn't seem to suffer like so many terminally ill people do."

Neither Ione nor Mary Anne ever lost sight of who Ione was. Many aspects of her personality were able to shine through the dementia: "She was always upbeat. She never got depressed. Her assertiveness and her unique sense of humor remained.[30] Mom always knew her name. She would say, 'I'm Ione.'" Hearing Ione say her own name gave Mary Anne the gift of deep joy—the kind that brings tears to our eyes and reminds us that the Spirit lives *in between* people, even when their capacities decline.

Mary Anne was additionally surprised to discover that focusing on Ione's remaining capacities had the potential to bring them both joy. Early in her mother's illness, Mary Anne thought that people diagnosed with Alzheimer's didn't have any reason to live. As the illness progressed, however, she noticed that Ione was still experiencing and expressing enjoyment in the company of her family and in eating good food, particularly good desserts! Ione still liked connecting with and talking with others; her failing memory and cognition didn't prevent her from loving her family or enjoying her life in the present moment. She especially enjoyed feeling useful. Mary Anne gave Ione appropriate tasks so she could be successful and feel a sense of accomplishment and meaning: folding towels, snapping beans. Ione was pleased to complete these tasks, always asking for more. This desire to be of service is holy and deserves recognition. Mary Anne was able to see it and honor it. She felt great joy in seeing her mother feel proud and happy in her accomplishments, whatever they were.

As Ione's short-term memory failed, she began to talk more about the past, bringing Mary Anne a gift she never expected. Mary Anne's father had died when she was four, and the loss was so great for Ione that she couldn't talk about him without crying. As a result, Mary Anne knew very little about her father—until Alzheimer's took away some of Ione's memory and rekindled experiences from her past. Freed from the pain of losing her husband, she could talk about him without suffering. These were joyful conversations of discovery for Mary Anne.

The seizures and strokes that continued throughout Ione's long decline raised Mary Anne's awareness that we never know when death will come. During the time enough they had together, living always in the shadow of death's unpredictability,

Mary Anne became an assertive advocate for her mother at the nursing home. She insisted that Ione be cared for with dignity and with sensitivity to her individual needs, according to the plan of care created by the nursing home staff. Mary Anne was an inspiration for other family members. Through her example, she gave us courage to ask for similar quality care for our loved ones.

The depth of Mary Anne's attentiveness to Ione was touching. "I knew what Mom liked and I wanted things to be the way she liked them," she said. "If this was going to be her last day, I didn't want her to go to bed without her teeth brushed. I wanted the things that mattered to her to be attended to. It was about how well I knew her."

Through the experience of Alzheimer's, Mary Anne discovered how well she knew her mother, and how important it was to know herself. Through Ione's illness and death, Mary Anne found her faith in both God and herself increasing. "I know I can handle more now—without crumbling—than I ever thought I could."

Mary Anne deeply mourned the loss of her mother when she died in 2008, but while Ione was alive, Mary Anne cherished every moment they had together. "Although our relationship was not the same, I never felt as if I had lost Mom. In some ways dementia deepened our connection. Because of Mom's vulnerability, I felt closer to her than I ever had, and my love and respect for her was even greater because of what she was going through."

Trust was one aspect of their relationship that deepened. In certain stages of their disease, people with dementia often become fearful, almost paranoid. Sometimes when Ione's husband Ed would try to give her medication, she would refuse and become very upset. She was convinced that he was trying to poison her. Ed quickly learned that he could call Mary Anne, whose reassuring voice would tell Ione that the pills were safe and that Ed was trying to help her. Ione would hang up the phone and cooperatively take her pills. Sometimes at night, Ione would wake up in utter distress because she couldn't find her kids. Again, Ed learned quickly to call Mary Anne, who, awakened from her sleep, would calm Ione. With her sleepy but familiar voice, Mary Anne was able to relieve her mother's anxiety by saying, "Don't worry, Mom, the kids are all here, and I'm taking good care of them." Then they could all sleep in peace.

"Mom having dementia wasn't the best thing," Mary Anne admits. "It wasn't something we would ever have chosen, but because Mom had this deep level of trust in me, I was able to be content with the situation. It was such a privilege to be *the* trusted person in Mom's life, and it made me want to be worthy of her trust."

Time Enough for Joy

Mom's nursing home offered the Catholic Mass in their chapel every day for the residents. After I moved to Iowa, it took a number of months for me to figure out that Mom attended Mass only when I accompanied her, usually on Sundays. Although the nursing home provided this religious ritual, residents who couldn't say yes when asked if they wanted to go to Mass, or couldn't remember the time and place, and then get themselves to the chapel on time, were taken only when their families had made prior arrangements.

My teachers and guides had impressed upon me that persons with Alzheimer's can only initiate activities in ways consistent with their potential.[31] Their lack of initiating, however, doesn't mean that they don't want to participate in an activity. There was no doubt that Mom wanted to attend Mass whenever it was offered. Through her own words, actions, and initiative—when she still had the capacity to assert her own will—Mom communicated to me that Mass was important to her. During our weeks together in 2004, Mom gathered up her purse every morning, informing me that it was Sunday and time for the 11:00 Mass. Before I realized that Mom needed to be supervised, she would leave the house without my knowledge. At first, I would panic when I noticed she was gone. My panic subsided, however, as soon as I figured out she would *always* be found two blocks away, at church.

Mom's ability to remember and appreciate her lifelong religious rituals was surviving the destruction of Alzheimer's. She remembered the rosary, which she could also participate in regularly at the nursing home, upon request. At Mass, she looked intently at the prayer book, which I helped her to hold. She especially enjoyed turning the pages when I cued her that it was time. I'm quite sure the familiar words and music of the service were reassuring, as were the taste and texture of the communion wafer. The sight of the priest at the altar, the vestments, the candles, and the shiny chalices filled with water and wine all mesmerized her.

The Sunday Mass at the nursing home was always crowded to capacity with residents, many in wheelchairs, and a few visiting family members. During the first years after I moved to Iowa, Mom and I proudly walked together to the front of the chapel where Mom could see everything clearly. As her disease progressed and she needed to use a wheelchair for any distance, we sat in the back of the chapel and became part of the sea of others in wheelchairs. Throughout the service, I slowly rolled Mom's chair back and forth in a rocking motion, adding a sense of soothing and comfort to her experience.

As I observed the priest saying Mass, I wondered what it was like for him to prepare a daily homily and preside over a service at which many of his congregants were asleep and most couldn't comprehend his interpretation of the scriptures or the sanctity of the Eucharist. One day I asked him about this, and he replied, "Whenever two or more are gathered in God's name, there is love." The condition of those in attendance didn't matter to Father Ron. The presence of the residents, who would receive what they could receive; the compassion he felt for "his people"; and the faithful leading of the religious ritual he had been ordained to perform—these were what mattered to him.

If Mom didn't attend Mass, she was in her room alone and sleepy. Sometimes the aides turned on her TV, but rarely was she engaged. And so Mass offered ritual and community, both of which were important and meaningful to Mom and her neighbors. Although Catholicism was no longer my chosen religious tradition, I started taking Mom to Mass so she would have something to do besides sit in her room in isolation. Because I believed this activity was meaningful for her, I had deliberately made it a priority in my life. Quite unexpectedly, however, this ritual had also become meaningful for me. It was such a surprise one Sunday morning to realize that I was really looking forward to attending Mass with Mom.

When we left Mass, I always felt deeply connected to Mom and the other residents, spiritually enriched, and forever enlightened about the journey of life. It seemed that something astonishing often happened at this Mass, and this possibility kept me alert. One Sunday in the middle of the Mass, a woman in a wheelchair shouted out repeatedly, "Where am I? Why am I here? I don't know what I'm doing here!" I was awakened in the moment by the important existential questions this woman was asking. Why have I been created? Why am I here? These are the most mysterious questions in life, and I had often thought about them myself. Why am I in Iowa? Why am I on earth? This wise woman reminded me to refresh my inquiry.

No one had rushed in to shush the inquiring woman or whisk her out of the chapel for creating a disturbance, and I was so pleased by this. It was a "come as you are, however you are" kind of Mass, and everyone was accepted. Imperfections and irregularities were welcomed, and I felt that I fit right in. Never before, or since, has a church service been so meaningful to me.

Because it was such enjoyable and enlightening quality time together, I often tried to arrange my schedule so Mom and I could attend Mass together on weekdays. On Mondays and Wednesdays after Mass, an exercise class was held in the large space outside the chapel. The class leader, Dee, was a woman in her eighties. She noticed me at Mass with Mom and kept inviting us to join her class. I knew the class content was way beyond Mom's abilities, but continually rejecting Dee's gracious invitation wasn't feeling good to me. So one Wednesday, we stayed. Mom couldn't possibly respond to or keep up with the instructions, but I quickly realized that I could assist her. I moved her arms and legs, tapped her feet, stretched her neck and shoulders, and moved from side to side so she would follow me with her eyes. The exercises were set to music and included a combination of old songs such as "My Wild Irish Rose" and the theme from *The Mickey Mouse Club*; more modern songs with movements, such as "YMCA" (we shaped our bodies into the letters) and the "Macarena," inspiring songs like "I Believe I Can Fly," and my personal favorite, which was just for fun, the "Chicken Dance." It was a marvelous way to take care of Mom's body, to increase her circulation, and to keep her muscles moving. And I got a real workout too, especially while lifting and rotating her legs. Filled with delight during this class, we smiled, laughed, danced, and waved batons with long, flowing, colorful scarves attached to the ends. For forty minutes, Alzheimer's was forgotten, and movement, joy, and deep connection filled our present moments.

Instantly, this activity caught fire in my soul, and I deliberately rearranged my schedule so Mom and I could attend the exercise class every Monday and Wednesday, in addition to Mass, if she felt well enough. For me, this experience seemed like the exercise, socialization, and connection sought by mothers who attend "Mommy and Me" classes with their infants and toddlers. It was fun, energizing, and purposeful. The class provided a full-body workout for Mom, comparable to thirty to forty minutes of physical therapy, gave us both physical and social contact, and created a mother-daughter bonding experience beyond any expectations. At this class, I discovered that play is vital to the soul.

Alzheimer's gave Mom and me more time together, and the exercise class gave us an opportunity to bond through joyful experience. I concluded that nursing homes and senior centers should start advertising exercise (dance, movement, or recreation) classes for aging parents and adult children and really encourage the daughters and sons to come and assist their parents. In my opinion, we adult children, as well as persons with Alzheimer's, can all use a little more high-energy fun in our lives. And there it was—every Monday and Wednesday—just waiting for Mommy and me.

Time Enough for Healing

Carl and I had been ministerial colleagues since the early 1990s, and we had lived in the same geographical area for nearly twenty years. However, my 2003 discovery of his mother's poem "The Wind of the Spirit"[32] was actually the seed of our friendship. A few years later, we connected more deeply in a peer group of spiritual directors, and our friendship grew. When I began the journey through Alzheimer's with my mother, however, and learned that Carl and Myra had walked this path before us, an enduring, supportive friendship blossomed.

When I asked Carl to participate in my exploration of the blessings caregivers receive from their loved ones with Alzheimer's, he agreed. He did not agree, however, with my premise that there were blessings to be found anywhere near Alzheimer's disease. He explained that, throughout Myra's decline, he experienced "terrible pain in seeing her in pain and not being able to change things. It was awful for her, awful for me." Carl claimed there were no moments of joy for him.

While preparing for our meeting to talk about his Alzheimer's experiences, Carl resurrected his journals from the time of his mother's illness as well as his files about her care and her life in various facilities. As he reviewed these old documents, Carl unearthed surprising blessings that had been there all along, just waiting to be discovered. Through the questions I posed to Carl, and through his own reflections on his feelings and experiences during his mother's illness and beyond, he was able to see the journey with his mother differently. He saw how painful this time was for him. He also saw, however, that his mother's diminishment was a call to love. "It was a call I could *not* say no to." "Widen your hearts to us, O Corinthians,"[33] Carl eloquently quoted the apostle Paul's second letter. Then he said, "Mom taught me to widen my heart."

Ten years after his mother's death, as Carl read and reread his journals with fresh eyes and a now-widened heart, he realized that his call and the call to many others caring for parents with Alzheimer's is "a precious and unique experience that will be with us for the rest of our lives." As Myra's abilities diminished and Carl's caregiving responsibilities increased, he experienced a crisis fraught with stress and spiritual decline. Finally realizing that he couldn't neglect his own welfare, Carl began to pray as never before. Instead of reciting the prayers he had learned from his parents in childhood, he sat each morning with his God, pouring his heart out, and asking for help to get through the day. Carl quickly understood that this kind of prayer is not just for a crisis. "This is for a lifetime," he said.

Although Carl and Myra had a "warmly cordial relationship" throughout his life, they were not close. Carl's parents were very busy Chinese missionaries, and he and four of his five siblings were raised in China by an *amah* from infancy through childhood. "In retrospect," Carl said, "caring for Mother was an experience of resolving a distance I had always felt with her, and I sensed she felt with me. There was not hostility between us. There was distance."

Throughout Myra's illness, Carl grieved. Upon reflection, he realized that his grief went deeper than the loss of his mother to Alzheimer's and ultimately death: "I had a fear of losing a relationship with my mother that I never really had. And so I wasn't grieving just the loss of our actual relationship. I was grieving the loss of a relationship we never had, and now could never, would never have." Or so he feared at the time.

Carl's journal from a year after Myra's death chronicled his realization of how affectionate he had become with his mother during the course of Alzheimer's. He realized that an intimacy they had never before shared had grown between them during those years of her diminishment: "Before Mother's illness, I always gave her a ritual hug when I came and left. We talked about church, sermons, who was doing what. We didn't talk relationships." With reflection, Carl was able to recall many moments of pleasure and connection with Myra during her illness: "I would pray with Mom, sing to her, read to her, and tell her what was happening. During her illness, I felt *deep* pleasure in her company, and *deep* affection toward her. I talked warmly with her. I *felt* I was giving her love. I sat close to her and put my arm around her. I put my head close to her—cheek to cheek. I called her 'Little Mother.' And when I fed her, I always gave her the ice cream first!"

Myra was bedridden and curled into the fetal position for two and a half years before she died. She ate, eliminated, breathed, and slept. Despairing family members repeatedly queried each other and medical professionals, "Why is she still living?" And when she finally did die, Carl's first words when he heard were, "Oh, thank God."

It took more than a decade and an inquiring colleague to spur Carl into reflection about his mother's illness and the years he journeyed with her. In this reflection, he discovered that, in spite of the losses from Alzheimer's, her life had increasing value to him. "What made Mom's life of great value to me was the relationship I had with her during her illness, and what

I was learning—even though I didn't know I was learning." Carl laughed as he continued, "A lesson is a lesson whether you know it or not!"

In the time enough Alzheimer's disease gave to Carl and Myra, Carl had the opportunity to show his mother the love he felt he never received from her. In doing this, he said, "I healed myself."

Like the Monarch butterflies, we rely on our own instincts and the instincts of our companions for guidance on the journey home. We help each other to get there with dignity by offering encouragement, support, comfort, companionship . . . and love. Although persons with Alzheimer's may not remember cognitively that they are on the journey home, they remember with their instincts and with their hearts. And in their hearts, they remember what will help them most along the way. They remember love.

Choose love. There is *always* time enough for love.

The Last Word

I have put off writing about my last experiences with Mom. I knew it would open that wound of missing her. I would relive the pain of losing my mother bit by bit through Alzheimer's disease, and then completely losing her through death.

Over many days, procrastination was my companion. But as I began to write, I realized that remembering and revering all of our moments together, including those of loss and pain, would be the path to accessing and integrating the joy and love we shared. Writing was how I could honor my mother as my important companion, teacher, and guide through Alzheimer's disease, through death, and into my new life.

As I consider last experiences, I share a poem written by Libbie Deverich Stoddard, who has been my close friend, colleague, and mentor for more than twenty years. She provided nurture for me when my mother wasn't able to offer enlightening words or comfort. It was Libbie who encouraged me to read *Learning to Speak Alzheimer's*, and when Mom's ability to speak was nearly extinguished, she once again offered guidance. Thinking of Mom and me, Libbie wrote this poem:

How Shall I . . . ?
I am losing words.

How shall I describe
the feeling of reaching toward,
reaching out, longing;
how shall I name
what I have loved
and do love,
still love: faces,
flowers, clouds, the long view
across prairie . . . and lake?

How will I greet you,
how will you know
you are greeted, loved,
and longed-for? Will you
believe me when it comes,
as it will,
that I speak without words,
and forget to hold my arms out
in embrace of you,
who are earth, and sky, and world;
how will I recognize
your embrace of me;
how will we continue
this life's long love,
when I have lost all words?

Mom and I lived each day with these questions, unsure of
the answers, but open to finding them.

The hundreds of young women working in Mom's nursing
home were having babies. The older women's daughters were
having babies. Through many pregnancies, many births, and
many babies' visits to Mom's floor, I witnessed the process of
life beginning, while at the same moment in time, I was also

witnessing the process of life ending.

When a baby is expected, we celebrate the first movement inside the womb, placing curious, delighted hands on the mother's growing belly. We anticipate that awe-inspiring moment of birth, sharing each new development with amazement and joy. The sonograms are passed around the lunch table. Detailed birth stories are gaily shared. There are stories about the child's first breath, signaled by the first cry. Thus begins the long list of firsts to be recognized and celebrated: first smile, first word, first step . . .

Through all of these stories of firsts, I found myself comparing the attention lavished on children at the beginning of life with the withdrawal of attention from elders at the end of life. We anticipate and celebrate the first word. Parents want to be present when that first precious word is spoken, and the nursing home's working moms lamented with misery if they missed this or any other firsts. Their instinct to love almost demanded that they be present to witness that first miraculous word.

What about the last step? The last word? The last smile? What about the continuing growth process that leads us to death *from* this life instead of to birth *into* this life?

Carl noticed a distinction between joy and pleasure during the journey through Alzheimer's with his mother Myra. He didn't feel joy with his mother because exuberance was not present. New mothers are, indeed, often exuberant, uninhibitedly enthusiastic. Carl recognized, however, that he did feel pleasure and satisfaction in his mother's presence. Similarly, the last step, the last word, the last smile will perhaps not elicit enthusiastic feelings, but neither should they inspire absence. They could actually be the most valuable, the most memorable, the most healing, and the most surprisingly inspiring moments of our lives.

The process of dying to this life is represented by our natural growth into "lasts." These amazing expressions of this natural process deserve honor and respect. Overcoming our fear of mortality and dread of Alzheimer's will allow us to experience the awe-inspiring potential for transformation. Mom's last word embodied this potential.

The last word I heard Mom speak was on my birthday during the summer of 2007. For Mother's Day that year, I had sent her a framed picture of us taken in the front yard of our house when I was two months old. She was holding me. Her advocate at the nursing home wrote me a note sharing Mom's reaction to the photo. "I could tell she enjoyed it," the advocate wrote, "as her eyes were on the picture for a good long time while holding it." By the time my birthday arrived in August of that year, I was with Mom in Iowa. I took the picture down from the wall in her room and showed it to her. Mom immediately took it from me and held it tightly with both hands. She looked at me, then at the baby in the picture. These were long, intent gazes. Mom looked at me again, her inquiring blue eyes meeting my receptive blue eyes. Then she clearly said my name: "Jade."

Until that moment, I wasn't sure if Mom realized I was her daughter. Her last word, however, connecting me to the baby picture, told me that she knew I belonged to her. Even in the later stages of Alzheimer's, some part of Mom's brain could still make a relational connection, and with her remaining capacity, she spoke one last word so that I would know she recognized me.

What a gift I was given, the forever cherished memory of hearing my mother's last word! Of course, I didn't know at the time that it would be her last word. But there were even greater gifts to be received. On the surface, there was the heart-opening gift of knowing that Mom's last word was my name and that she knew me. But on a deeper level, this one word strengthened my faith in my mission. Mom knew who I was. She knew I was there with her on this journey. I hoped, believed, that in knowing her daughter, Jade, was with her, Mom felt safe, secure,

comforted, and loved as she walked deeper into the mystery of
Alzheimer's disease on her way home.

When Libbie sent her poem to me, I didn't know the answer to
"How Shall I . . . ?" It was one of those questions whose answer,
according to poet Rainer Maria Rilke, must be lived into:

> I beg you . . . to have patience with everything unsolved
> in your heart and try to love the *questions themselves* as
> if they were locked rooms or books written in a very
> foreign language. Don't search for the answers, which
> could not be given to you now because you would not
> be able to live them. And the point is, to live everything.
> *Live* the questions now. Perhaps then, someday far in the
> future, you will gradually, without even noticing it, live
> your way into the answer.[34]

Rilke's wisdom also reminded me to "take whatever comes
with great trust."[35] Encouraged, I walked on with Mom, trusting that together we would discover how her love and her
needs would be communicated. Along the way, professionals in
the field of Alzheimer's care gave me insights. At an Alzheimer's
conference, I learned from speech and language pathologist
Michelle Bourgeois that persons with Alzheimer's are *attempting* to communicate. As we open our ears and eyes to a new
type of communication process, we may be surprised by the
possibilities that remain.[36] Stephan Millett identifies persons
with Alzheimer's as "semiotic subjects,"[37] indicating that they
are proficient at using signs and symbols for communication
purposes. We must learn to translate.

Later that summer, Mom demonstrated one way we would
live into the answer of "How Shall I . . . ?" On a Saturday morning, two of my cousins came from out of town to see Mom
and me. John, a psychiatrist living in California, was visiting his

sister Lucy, who lived about a hundred miles from Dubuque. Although Mom had not seen them for a few years, she seemed to recognize their voices right away. Knowing how much Mom loved this duo and how much she enjoyed hugging, I helped her to stand up from her recliner chair. John and Lucy lined up to give Mom a hug, and I stepped out of the way, partly sitting, partly leaning against the heating and air conditioning unit in her room. First Lucy and then John: Mom hugged them and she smiled. Then, taking me completely by surprise, she turned around, facing me. She walked a few steps toward me and opened her arms, inviting me into the best hug ever. She smiled. I was teary. Then, realizing that Mom had just demonstrated her remaining ability to initiate and express affection, I smiled, and we hugged and laughed together in a moment of pure joy.

My earliest teacher about Alzheimer's, Joanne Koenig Coste, writes, "The emotion behind the failing words is far more important than the words themselves, and needs to be validated. Assume the patient can still register feelings that matter."[38] Mom showed me how true this was.

While I was wondering about how Mom and I would communicate without words, I encountered the work of Stephen Levine, Buddhist teacher, groundbreaking practitioner and author in the field of loss, dying, and grief, and colleague of Dr. Elisabeth Kübler-Ross, the psychiatrist and pioneer in the field of death and dying who developed the Five Stages of Grief model. Levine reminded me that, "from the day we are born, we communicate without language."[39] In their book *Who Dies? An Investigation of Conscious Living and Conscious Dying*, Stephen and Ondrea Levine brought to my attention a term that helped me understand and embrace the living answer to how Mom and I could communicate when her words were lost: *heart speech*. Describing heart speech as words and feelings arising within us that may or may not be audibly expressed,

Stephen Levine first used this phrase to describe a style of communicating through presence and intuition with people in comas and people who are close to death. As he sat at bedsides, silently experiencing and expressing understanding and compassion, restless patients would become calm, tears would clear, eyes would meet in knowing awareness, and peace would enter the space. Levine describes his experience as sitting quietly and sending love and understanding through his heart. He does not claim that the ill or dying person picked up the silent words in his heart through some kind of telepathy; however, he believes and experienced that the "attitude of love and care generated an acceptance of the moment" that brought forth an atmosphere of peacefulness.[40]

When the Levines first began implementing their skillful practice of heart-speech in hospitals and hospices in the 1970s and 1980s, many of the nurses began to try it. They "said it changed their relationships to many of their patients and their painful job in general. They had another tool to open to another, and perhaps transmit that openness." Other nurses came forward to express "how wonderful it was to hear someone speak of a technique that they had intuitively been employing for some time."[41]

Through his decades of experience in the world of death and dying, Levine concludes that people who may seem disengaged and unresponsive, especially as their verbal abilities decline—"often are reachable through heart speech and . . . trust in the depth of our connection as human beings."[42] My own trust in my connection with Mom inspired me to to believe that communicating with her in deep and meaningful ways was still possible.

My young friend Crystal visits regularly with her aunt, who has dementia and lives in a nursing home. She naturally discovered heart speech and has explained to me that this kind of communication is neither mysterious nor complicated. She simply sits with her Aunt Grace, who is very confused in her recollections and her speaking. In her aunt's presence, Crystal consistently maintains the attitude that it's OK for Grace to be confused. Approaching confusion with an attitude of acceptance relieves the pressure on the person with Alzheimer's to get it right.

Earlier in my life's journey, I worked in human resources for a large financial institution. My job included communication training for managers. There I learned that a required aspect of effective communication is reception. For communication to actually take place, the message must be received. I taught managers how to effectively encode their messages so their communications would have a better chance of being received and understood by their employees.

Now that Mom had lost all words, the writings of Allen Power, Pierre Parenteau, and Stephen and Ondrea Levine were teaching me how to communicate with her—to both send messages and to receive messages so that our process of communicating would be effective. They respectively recommended curiosity, intuition, and heart speech.[43] St. Benedict offered me additional guidance: "Attend with the ear of your heart."[44]

Mom was already proficient in heart speech, as is often the case with persons who are dying and non-verbal, and/or living with more active intuitive right brain function due to stroke or disease. Stephen Levine writes, "Somehow, it seems, many who are seriously ill are sensitive to such deep touching."[45] I was the one who needed to learn. At first, I tried being chatty with Mom, telling her the details of my day. She sat quietly and without expression through this process, which felt somehow empty to me. It seemed that reception was missing, and being chatty quickly became tiring and dull for me. I assume it had the same effect on Mom. She did, however, respond joyfully to the sound of my voice, so I often read and sang to her. When

I talked to her, I used simple words and phrases with a positive tone and musical inflection. I intentionally maintained physical contact with her during our interactions. My words were always affectionate and encouraging, and my touch was tender and loving. I was sending Mom the feelings in my heart.[46]

When I began to use words more sparingly, I felt energized by my interactions with Mom, which would not be surprising to Stephen Levine. He already knows that the intuitive process of heart speech, which sends truth and love directly from one heart to another, is "of considerable value to the sender of such wholehearted blessings."[47]

Levine's description of heart speech as "meeting deeply in the heart" expressly identifies this kind of communication as relational and reinforces the idea of being carepartners with persons with Alzheimer's. We connect with "another silently, intuitively, feeling as one might when singing a child to sleep. We speak into another's heart as an expansion of our own continued healing."[48] Persons with Alzheimer's are communicating with heart speech all the time. Although they "have lost all words," and can no longer comprehend all of our words, they can transmit and receive the attitude of love and care and acceptance.

Once I had learned to communicate with Mom using heart speech, we sent each other reciprocal messages of love, care, and acceptance every day, often through a look or a smile or a touch. Practicing this kind of communication for over three years, I came to realize and benefit from the deep healing it made possible. Stephen and Ondrea Levine explain, "When you speak from the heart you send love, not your needs or desires for people to be any way other than they are."[49] Stephen Levine reminds us, "We love what is instead of what might be,"[50] or in the circumstance of Alzheimer's disease—instead of what was. Loving what is can truly be a challenge for caregivers. I've heard family members say that they don't visit their relatives in decline because they want to remember their loved ones how they "used to be."

As Mom's disease progressed, our power struggle over my life choices had effortlessly ended. Those things I had done that hurt, frustrated, and angered her had silently been removed from her consciousness. It didn't seem to matter to Mom what I ate, what God I believed in, whether or not I avoided alcohol, if I had a schedule to keep, or if I wanted to meditate and exercise every day. She had lost the capacity to criticize, judge, and reject me, and in the absence of my fear of these capacities, I no longer felt defensive around her. I knew that Mom didn't exactly choose not to criticize, judge, or reject me. This knowledge, however, did not rob me of the experience of feeling totally, wholeheartedly accepted and loved by my mom, just exactly as I am, for the first time in my life. In Mom's present reality, I was her faithful, kind, loving, and protective companion. That's all that mattered to her. I felt so accepted and appreciated by her that the wound caused by knowing there were times she was not proud of me, times I had disappointed her, and times I was not who she wanted me to be began to heal in the presence of a mother who loved me—now.

My acceptance and my receptivity were also needed to activate the healing power of heart speech. Through my academic study of Alzheimer's and my personal experiences and observations, I had learned about the process of decline determined by Mom's disease, and I had fully accepted her increasing limitations. While learning and accepting, I had developed realistic expectations of Mom. I had completely let go of expecting her to be the kind of mother I had always wanted, and I accepted the kind of mother she had now become. Once I did so, I was able to notice that she had, in many ways, become the mother I needed.

The Sufi poet Rumi had informed me years earlier about the transformation and healing that are possible through this kind of acceptance.

Learn the alchemy True Human Beings know:
The moment you accept what troubles you've been given,
the door opens.[51]

My acceptance and my now realistic expectations of Mom
had opened the door for me to recognize her as the one person
in the world who could never disappoint me. I didn't expect,
demand, or want her to be anyone other than who she was
at each moment. I gracefully and gratefully received what she
could give, and I didn't ask for or need more.

From this new perspective, I could see how much Mom was
still able to give me, including important things that a daughter needs from her mother. Because Mom's diminished capacities kept her in one place all the time—her nursing home—I
received the gift of being able to trust that she would always be
available and receptive to me whenever I needed my mom, like
when I was sad or stressed and needed a hug or a smile from
someone who cared. She was always happy to see me, always.
She was an attentive audience whenever I needed to talk, never
interrupting me and hijacking the conversation (the pattern
she had perpetuated throughout my life). And she let me know
how important I was to her, through looks, smiles, touches, and
sounds—her perfect version of heart speech.

Even though she perhaps lacked the ability to formulate an
intention to mother me in these ways, Mom's presence still gave
me the experience of being mothered. Sometimes I actually sat
on her lap. Although I weighed less than a hundred pounds and
Mom was still quite robust at the time, I always kept one foot
on the floor, making sure to hold most of my weight off her. I
also used this foot to rock the wheelchair slowly back and forth.
Mom had her arms tightly around me, and I imitated the voice
of her baby doll, softly saying, "Mama, Mama." I was inspired
to say these words often, believing they were a comfort, believing that if Mom could speak, she would be saying, "Mama,

Mama," to me. I'm not sure which one of us was healed more by what felt like an experience of mutual mothering. The look on Mom's face at these times seemed peaceful and content. This deep connection between us was made possible by the grace of her diminishment and her increasing ability to experience the world by functioning and communicating through the intuitive, emotional right side of her brain.[52] These changes had inspired us both to open our hearts to the flow of love. We had both grown into the most accepting, most loving, and most nonjudgmental persons we had ever been.

Although Alzheimer's was the catalyst for the changes within us and the deep connection growing between us, our acceptance of and love for each other was no less real or profound. What Mom gave me, and what she received from me, was enough to create a deep and strong bond that we both recognized and cherished.

Many family members suffer from believing that Alzheimer's is a kind of death before death, feeling that their loved ones with Alzheimer's are already gone. I didn't experience this particular suffering because I recognized so many signs of life through Mom's efforts at self-expression. I later learned that, throughout the human development process, we all, including persons with Alzheimer's, possess an innate drive to maximize our potential.[53]

At the end of my seven-week visit during the summer of 2007, I returned to Boston for a semester of school and to make arrangements for moving to Iowa. In October, Mom's social worker informed me that she had a bad cold, was weak, and wasn't walking. They speculated that this would mark the end of her ability to get out of the wheelchair, and I was sure I had accompanied Mom on some of her last steps. She surprised everyone, however, by expressing her potential. By the time I returned in December, she was walking again!

Mom had always been physically active, doing yard work, shoveling snow, painting the exterior of her house by herself, and walking a mile to and from work every day for more than twenty years. Knowing that being active was important to her, I wanted to preserve her physical abilities and help her continue to find enjoyment in using her body for as long as possible. A year after I moved to Iowa, a hospice physician informed me that I had been successful. Mom had been a hospice patient for a year, and was being "graduated." Not only had she not died but, even as Alzheimer's had predictably progressed, her physical condition and capabilities had improved. The doctor remarked that, given the progression of her disease, now in the end stage, Mom would have been bedridden and completely helpless if I hadn't been there every day, walking with her, engaging her in activities, helping her maintain her skills (such as feeding herself), and giving her loving attention. I hadn't realized that my efforts to enhance Mom's quality of life would support her desire to maximize her potential in such a significant way.

Everyone was amazed by Mom's remaining capabilities. A few times during the last years of her life, she was hospitalized for infections. Because I didn't want her to forget how to walk, each time I requested a physical therapist to come daily to help Mom get out of bed and walk with her. "Seriously?" the nurses always asked. "Seriously," I replied. And when Mom walked and smiled wide at them, the very surprised nurses instantly fell in love with her. Heart speech was working its magic.

As the disease progressed and Mom no longer qualified for physical therapy or rehabilitation programs offered by the nursing home, according to Medicare definitions, we were on our own. I asked for and received permission from the nursing home to take Mom to the physical therapy room and use some of their equipment. There were toys for hand dexterity and strength, balls for catching and throwing, and our favorite, the portable stairs. I would push this big platform into the middle of the room and position Mom facing the stairs going up. I stood on the other side of the up and then down stairs and asked her to come to me. At first, she needed coaching about holding the rails, lifting her right leg, pulling herself up, and lifting her left leg. And then, up she went. She was better going up than going down, but if I asked her to look at me, instead of the steps, she sailed down the three steps with ease. We practiced stairs on Sundays after Mass while most other residents sat alone in their rooms waiting for lunch. Mom's legs got stronger, she walked confidently without assistance, and she so enjoyed the big hug waiting for her at the end of the stair climbing.

One day, Mom and I were taking a ride in the nursing home minibus to see the sights around town. Bus rides always ended with an ice-cream cone from the Dairy Queen, and this was a treat for all the residents. Mom loved the bus! She even enjoyed the rides when the destination was the doctor's office. During the months I was away coordinating my move, the staff transferred Mom into the bus by having her sit in a wheel-chair and then ride up on the mechanical lift. I agreed to their process. As we walked out the front door toward the waiting wheelchair, Mom let go of my hand and walked with inten-tion directly toward the open door of the bus. She had seen the stairs! Without any assistance or direction, she put both hands on the rails and lifted her right foot onto the first step. There she paused. I'm sure the staff was thinking, "Oh no. What do we do now?" I went and stood behind her, coaching her as I had in the physical therapy room: "Pull yourself up with your arms, and lift your left leg up." She followed this instruction and climbed the rest on her own. Up all the steps she went into the bus. The staff and the residents already on the bus applauded. Mom radiated smiles and pride!

Eventually, our stair climbing practice ceased. One Sunday, Mom could no longer climb down the stairs. She was stuck at the top, seeming to panic about what to do. Perhaps her panic was a reflection of my own. I didn't want to leave her alone, fearing she would move and fall, but I needed to get help. So I asked Mom clearly to stand still and wait for me to get back. Thankfully, she did. I rushed out and found a nursing aide, who helped me to get Mom down the steps. But Mom was scared, a clear indication that the stair-climbing activity was now beyond her ability. Then came the time when walking to and from the dining room was too exhausting, then she could no longer walk with just one person assisting her, then she could walk only to the door of her room, and then, about a week before she died, she could no longer stand on her own. Through observation and acceptance of Mom's decline, I adjusted my expectations according to her abilities.

The aides at the nursing home who were Mom's most beloved caregivers also witnessed Mom's drive to maximize her physical potential. In the telling of the endearing stories of her accomplishments, we all became closer. As Mom's hands became more constricted and clenched, the occupational thera- pist brought palm guards to keep her fingernails from damag- ing her palms. One day, her aide Alexis was trying to get Mom to relax her hands and open her fingers enough to put on the palm guards. Trying to get Mom's clenched fists to open was challenging and time consuming, and the aides needed to be careful to avoid hurting her fingers. The occupational therapist had taught us all how to do the necessary hand massage, but this took a long time. Having other tasks to do, Alexis became exas- perated and finally wailed, "Oh, come on, Jeanne. Help me out here. Open up your fingers." And open them she did. No one had thought to ask Mom to do this. She opened them every day after this, very slowly, upon request.

Two weeks before Mom died, she caught a cold and her breathing was labored. We went briefly to the emergency room for a breathing treatment to make her more comfortable. The ER staff at the hospital was always remarkably kind to Mom.

They treated her as they would any other patient, which, sadly, isn't consistently the case with medical and hospital personnel encountering persons with dementia. Even though Mom was severely impaired by Alzheimer's and clearly not feeling well during the last ER visit, she was still able to surprise the doctor. The nurse was taking Mom's blood pressure from her left arm, and Mom was watching her intently. The doctor stood on Mom's right side, and from this position, with her looking away from him, he said her name, "Jeanne." Slowly, she turned her head, looked right at him, and smiled. I could see the surprise in his eyes, which matched his exclamation. "Wow!" he said.

All persons with Alzheimer's have the drive to maximize their remaining potential, and there will be countless opportunities for caregivers to nurture that drive. We just have to closely and carefully attend with the ears and eyes of our hearts, and give them chances to surprise us.

Mom and I communicated through heart speech until she drew her last breath. She was in the hospital over the Thanksgiving weekend, and although she recovered from the condition that took her there, I knew we were at the doorsill of her departure from this world. Before we left for the nursing home, we waited together for the van to come for us. We sat quietly holding hands, looking out the window. During this contemplative time, I realized that it would be helpful to know what Mom needed from me to get ready for her journey into the next life.

When I got home that night, I contacted a local holistic healer who I experienced as an intuitive and loving person. I asked her to come and sit with Mom, to see if she could receive any clarity about what else Mom might need from me at this time. The healer said she was open to doing this but didn't feel she was the right person. Feeling let down at a time of need,

I was upset. I didn't feel confident in my own intuition about something this important, so I tried to find someone else in nearby Madison, Wisconsin, without success.

Almost rebelliously, I decided to do it myself. I put on our favorite soft music. I held Mom's hand and asked her through heart speech, "What do you need, Mom, to get ready to go?" Intuitively, I received her reply: "I need to feel wanted." Given Mom's life story of abandonment, this reply didn't surprise me at all.

From that day until the moment she died, I let Mom know with my words and my actions that I loved taking care of her, loved being with her, and wanted her to be a part of my life. I didn't want to confuse her or delay her journey, however, so I also let her know that Jesus wanted her too, and that it was OK to go to him.

On Christmas Eve, while I was brushing her teeth, Mom looked up at me with eyes overflowing with trust. I was so moved that I couldn't hold her gaze. I gathered her up into my arms and held her close, telling her with my heart that I would do my best to be worthy of her trust.

Two days later, I asked her again what she needed. I sensed her reply: "Will you stay and wait with me?" I felt chills throughout my body. Her request reminded me of Jesus' request of Peter, James, and John as he prayed in the Garden of Gethsemane for the cup of suffering to be taken away from him. Jesus "began to be distressed and agitated. And said to them, 'I am deeply grieved, even to death; remain here, and keep awake.'"[54] Mom was confirming the insight of Thibault and Morgan: When persons with Alzheimer's are dying, nothing is more important "than family members sitting with them, holding their hands, and praying with them as their spirits leave this world for the next."[55]

"Of course, Mom," my heart replied to hers. "I promise I will stay and wait with you." I reassured her of this every day with my words as well as my presence.

I sent a note to the holistic healer, thanking her for paying attention to her hesitancy to help me. I was pleased to let her know that the right person to listen to Mom was me.

Eight days later, I arrived at the nursing home in the morning. Mom looked beautiful, wearing the snowflake turtleneck I had given her for her birthday. Her hair was brushed and gleaming. Colorful clips decorated her hair, and a white beaded necklace completed her ensemble. We hugged and smiled, and off we went to exercise class. As I moved her arms and legs as instructed by the class leader, Mom was attentive and joyful. I helped her kick the colorful beach ball, and this made her smile. She ate a little that day, although she had made it clear a couple weeks earlier that food was no longer of interest. She was rapidly losing weight and becoming physically weak. She hadn't walked for a few days. But her eyes, her smile, and her spirit were shining brightly.

That night after dinner, I hugged Mom good night, and wheeled her to the bathtub room. At the door, I leaned over, looking deep into her eyes. The connection between us seemed so strong, I decided to see if she would give me a kiss, like she used to. (Months earlier, to my sadness, she had stopped responding to my request for a kiss.) I looked into her clear blue eyes, touched her hand, and slowly, clearly said, "Kiss." Like I used to, I demonstrated how to kiss. I put my finger to my lips, puckered, and kissed. Never losing eye contact, I said it again, "Kiss." Then I put my lips to her lips, and without hesitation, Mom kissed me good night. My eyes filled with tears; I hugged her again. "I love you, Mom. I want you to be with me."

It was hard to leave her that night. It was always hard to leave her. By the time I got home, I was elated. I felt high on life, literally. Mom and I had shared such a great day. I thought we would have many more. Maybe weeks. Maybe even a month or more together. I felt gloriously happy.

That night at 1:56 AM, my phone rang. I was awake instantly. The nurse on the other end of the phone recited incomprehensible medical details: heart rate, respiration, nonresponsive, mot-tling. "Should I come now?" I asked. "Yes," she replied. "Come now."

If ever I wanted to run away, it was now. How could I let her go? How could I be there witnessing her nonresponsive face, a death mask? I had never been with someone at the moment of death, and I was scared. Scared of death, scared of loss.

But I went. I kept my promise to Mom. I stayed, and I waited with her.

During the next fifty-eight hours, the web of relationality I had woven around Mom over the previous four years teemed with life, bringing guidance, companionship, and comfort. The nursing home carepartners were attentive to us both. Mom's dearest companion aide, Kathy, brought her a rosary bracelet to wear, and this bracelet is now my most cherished piece of jewelry. The hospice nurses were ever-present, monitoring and relieving Mom's perceived pain and distress, and consoling and guiding me through every aspect of this unfamiliar experience. Other family members with loved ones at the nursing home, our long-time companions, kept a vigil at Mom's door. The hospice chaplain, our cousin, Father Ron, and my pastoral friends, Rev. Diane and Marilyn, all came—and stayed. They prayed with us. Our hearts were touched, and our needs were filled.

Although Mom appeared unresponsive, our connection remained intact. We listened to music. I sang, prayed, and gently massaged her. I brushed her hair. The aides made space for me in her bed, and I snuggled close and held her, through the night and through the day. I tenderly stroked her face. She loved this most of all. I told her those truths still unsaid. Our hearts spoke of love and leaving.

Before I left Massachusetts, I had asked my spiritual director what she believed happened when someone died. She shared her recollection of one of Julian of Norwich's revelations. God told Julian not to fear death, because as we breathe our last breath out, God will come in upon it, and it will become one breath, the Breath of God.[56] I wanted to be with Mom, holding her for her last breath. I wanted to be next to God, breathing in, becoming part of that One Breath.

Three mornings after Mom kissed me good-bye, the hospice nurse—proficient in heart speech—told me that although Mom was torn about leaving her life with me and moving on, today would be her last day. I reassured Mom about my love, and about how much I wanted her to be in my life. "But Jesus wants you too. And it's OK to go to him now." For almost four years, I had been holding Mom's mortal being close, and now I needed to gently let her immortal being go. As I cried about having to let go of my mom, both my faith and my friends accompanied me tenderly across this threshold.

Two of Mom's relatives were coming from out of town to say good-bye. The hospice nurse, knowing my desire to be with Mom to receive her last breath, suggested that the others visit for only fifteen minutes. We all agreed, but I was distraught that Mom might die while I was away from her bedside. My friend Rev. Diane had attended at the bedsides of many dying people. She counseled me, "Just ask her to wait for you." I did this. I held Mom. I told her who was coming and that I would give them some time alone with her. "Wait for me to come back, please. Wait for me." Fifteen minutes later, I returned to Mom's bedside. Within a few minutes, her breathing became labored. Another fifteen minutes, and God and I became one with her last breath.

I wept. And then there was a vision of me walking with Mom on a long journey that led us to a dock stretching far out into the ocean. A large cruise ship was there—waiting. This was as far as I could go with Mom. She boarded, and as the ship sailed away, she waved good-bye to me from the deck. Then she was gone—out of my sight, off on this new adventure.

The last word. The last step. The last kiss. The last breath. The last good-bye.

I am so grateful and happy that I didn't miss them.

Looking Back,
Walking On

The person with dementia is eventually swept away,
while caregivers look back
and feel forever changed by their experiences.
— Stephen G. Post

On Thursday, January 6, 2011, my mom went on to her new life. At the same moment, we both stepped across the doorsills of new worlds.

Some who knew me through my caring of Mom remarked that she was my "whole world." That assessment wasn't exactly true since my life at the time was rich with purpose and meaningful relationships in addition to my care of Mom. What was and is true, however, is that Mom unquestionably became the love of my life. Most people, me included, look for this kind of fulfilling, intimate love in a romantic relationship. So imagine my surprise to find it in relationship with an old woman with Alzheimer's disease!

In many ways, Mom became my soul mate. Through Alzheimer's, she taught me the most important lessons for living —not at the beginning of my life, as one might expect of a parent, but at the end of hers. Mom taught me how to love with my whole heart, how to organize my life around what really matters, how to be a good person, and how to accept and appreciate what is. Mom gave me the opportunity, in David Steindl-Rast's words, to say a "limitless 'Yes' to everything as it is,"[1] including pain, loss, hardship, death, challenge, joy, discovery, surprise, healing, and love. Saying that limitless yes has been the most transforming experience of my life.

Catholic priest Ronald Rolheiser defines *soul mate* as "the one who takes you home."[2] If this is a true definition, perhaps I became Mom's soul mate as well. Tenderly, I carried her to the threshold of her new world. At Mom's funeral Mass, our cousin Father Ron delivered the homily. It wasn't until he spoke about how much Mom smiled when I was with her that I realized the actual purpose, and holiness, of my caregiving mission. He said, "When Jeanne was smiling, we knew she was not suffering either physical or emotional pain. Her smile indicated that she was going beyond herself, she was interested in her surroundings, and she was connecting with others."

I had come to be companion and advocate. I didn't realize that I would be enabling connection, maximizing potential, and relieving suffering. When Ron's words helped me to realize what I had done, I wept.

After Mom died, I missed caring for her. I missed (and still miss) the flowing love we shared every day. I miss her hugs and kisses, and her smile. I really miss her smile. In the midst of all the missing, however, I'm grateful to have had the time and opportunity to be Mom's companion and soul mate on the journey. Being the one to relieve her fear, pain, and suffering, even a bit, and being the one to take her home was such an honor.

Although I was her companion, Mom was really the guide on the journey. She was showing me, and all those she encountered along the way, how to live life and how to approach disability and death with acceptance, dignity, and joy in the remaining moments. Because of her cognitive decline, Mom's walk toward death seemed instinctual. She seemed to gracefully lean into it, without resistance, and hopefully without fear.

Looking back, I appreciate all those who encouraged me to pay attention to Mom's guidance and showed me how to allow Mom's wisdom about life and death to shine forth. Walking on, I realize that my experience of caring for Mom is still lighting my way. My learning in the school of life and love, by looking at the world through the lens of Alzheimer's disease, did not end when Mom died.

My world looks different now, and new . . .

Forgetting, Forgiving, Reconciling

Usually, when I'm presented with an important life lesson, or I'm working through an issue, my mind grasps what's happening long before my emotions do. Throughout my journey of personal and spiritual growth, my learning process has been what people commonly describe as "understanding it with my head, but not feeling it in my heart." The process for forgiving and reconciling with Mom happened in the opposite order—I felt it in my heart first. Although I recognized it at the time, I didn't have enough intellectual knowledge of true forgiveness to be able to articulate how it had actually happened.

A seminary course in the psychology and theology of forgiveness, which I took during Mom's last months of life, enlightened my understanding somewhat. But the final piece of the forgiveness puzzle came into my heart on Thanksgiving Day, almost ten months after Mom died. My Thanksgiving tradition includes writing a letter reviewing the highlights of my year to enclose with my holiday cards. In an effort to procrastinate from, or to prepare for—I'm not sure which—writing my highlights letter the year Mom died, I was looking through a file of old correspondence. Tucked away in that file were all the letters Mom had written to me on her teeny-tiny stationery in 2003 and 2004. I had not seen those letters, which chronicled her decline and expressed her appreciation for me, for eight or nine years. Accidently unearthing these treasures brought into full awareness my understanding of how and when the forgiveness and reconciliation that Mom and I experienced actually happened.

A few weeks after I officially relocated my life—including my car and all my belongings—from Boston to Iowa, Mom became very sick with the flu. It was serious, and she was accepted into the hospice program. On April 2, 2008, the nurse called me at 7 AM to report that Mom's fever had risen to 104 degrees. The hospice nurse and Mom's priest were called. I went to the nursing home immediately, climbed into Mom's bed, and snuggled next to her. I held her, rocked her, and put ice packs on her forehead. We all thought she would die that day, and I experienced the fullness of human sorrow.

I felt sorrow for the many ways Mom had harmed me, and for the close relationship I longed to have with her—that had never been. I felt sorrow because I had not been able to do more to protect Mom and nurture her during her time of need. I did what the system allowed me to do, and what my physical and emotional limits allowed me to do. I did my best, but oh, how I wished I could have done more for her. I felt sorrow because I never apologized to her, and she never apologized to me. I felt surprising sorrow because I had discovered how much I loved being with Mom, and all of what we now shared would be gone—too soon.

My friend's grandson, Gabriel, was born that day in the early morning hours. I got that news as I was rushing out the door to be at Mom's bedside. Gabriel begins. Mom ends. That's what I thought the day would be about. In the midst of this extraordinary day of birth and death, joy and sorrow, ordinary things were also happening. Mom and I listened to music as we often did. The birds outside were singing. The nursing home's cleaning woman vacuumed in the hallway outside Mom's door.

On that sorrowful, joyful, extraordinary, ordinary day, I suddenly felt the presence of God surrounding Mom and me. During one seemingly miraculous moment, which I was fortunate to notice in the midst of an intense swarm of emotions, I realized that I had forgiven my mother. It was as if her whole life flashed before my eyes and my heart suddenly knew and embraced her. I felt the life-filled breath of love flowing from my heart to her heart and back again. And I forgave her for everything.

Because this day of Mom's death was inevitable, people had asked me what I would do and how I would feel if Mom died shortly after I moved. In all my decision-making, I had to consider this possibility. My answer was, "I don't know." On that extraordinary day, however, I lived into knowing the answer to that question. If Mom had died only weeks after my cross-country relocation, I would have had no regrets about rearranging my priorities, letting go of my professional opportunities and aspirations, completely changing my life, and moving to be with her.

There I was, twelve hundred miles away from everything that was familiar to me, forgiving and loving one who had harmed me throughout my life, one who had betrayed and abandoned me during my times of great need. In spite of her failings, I was at her bedside. I had not forsaken her. My choices and my feelings in the context of our fractured relationship were hard to understand at the time, even for me. But, I knew one thing for certain: I had no regrets.

In my heart, the forgiveness I felt for Mom on that April morning was complete, arising spontaneously and effortlessly. It was just miraculously there, unbidden. I spoke of this experience often, and always with awe. Many reacted to my story of forgiveness with skepticism.

"Really? Forgiveness just happened?"

"Really," I would reply. "It just happened."

So it seemed, at the time.

Focusing attention, time, and energy on forgiving Mom for not protecting me from my father and for abandoning me when I most needed her help had not been a priority for me. Healing from the severe wounds of my childhood had appropriately been my focus. The writings of modern spiritual teachers and professionals working with childhood abuse survivors had urged me over the years not to forgive too quickly.[3] They describe the road leading to true forgiveness as long and arduous.[4] Later in my theological studies, I learned that numerous scholars echo this advice and this wisdom.[5]

During the last months and weeks of Mom's life, I studied and contemplated forgiveness in my seminary class. Challenged by the continual questioning of the skeptics, I was seeking to understand my spontaneous experience of forgiveness.

I was especially surprised to discover that my sense of forgiveness resonated with the understanding of this process as seen through the lens of the Jewish tradition, even though I had been raised in the tradition of Roman Catholicism. According to Professor Solomon Schimmel, a victim who has been unjustly injured is entitled to feel resentment "and the perpetrator has incurred a moral and/or legal debt to the victim, such as to apologize, make reparations or be punished." An abuser is not forgiven until reparation is made and forgiveness is formally requested from the injured person.[6] Judaism's interpretation was a comfort, letting me know that my anger and resentment toward my parents were justifiable, and that I was not a bad person for feeling as I did throughout much of my life. After all, my parents had not acknowledged my wounds and losses, nor had they asked for my forgiveness.

On the other hand, devout Christians are often taught that

forgiveness is a moral obligation—even if the abuser is unrepentant. Christians can, and must, forgive, because God is infinitely forgiving.

Although I didn't focus on forgiving Mom through the decades of my healing process before Alzheimer's touched my world, I intentionally kept communication open with her. Occasionally, I traveled to Iowa to visit her, truly hoping that one day she would see me, that she would recognize my hurt, be accountable, apologize, and make amends somehow. Unfortunately, our dueling priorities and lifestyles often collided, and after these visits with Mom it took weeks to recuperate and regain my sense of self-worth. "Why do you keep going there? Why do you put yourself through this?" friends asked. I wasn't sure. It seemed that, somewhere in my heart, a painful hope for forgiveness and reconciliation was springing eternally.

When Mom was diagnosed with Alzheimer's, my hope for an apology from her vanished, along with my hope for feeling forgiveness or having a meaningful relationship with her. I lamented, miserably, the fact that Mom would no longer be able to admit what had happened, to say she was sorry, or to make amends. Every possibility I could imagine for forgiveness and reconciliation was lost along with Mom's cognitive abilities. Hope was over.

As I grieved this loss of hope, one of my most important guides encouraged me to let go of expectations, and to remain open for surprise.

In the center of the Refiner's Fire of Alzheimer's, where the flames were burning away feelings I no longer needed and purifying my soul, I looked for insights about forgiveness. Observing Mom, myself, and other caregivers, especially my friend Mary Kay, from within the fire, I saw an intricate and complex web of impressions and emotions. I realized that our ideas about forgiveness are influenced by personal histories, misunderstood or misinterpreted theologies, and hearts longing for connection. In the context of Alzheimer's care within Mary Kay's life, Mom's life, and my own, several specific concepts related to forgiveness caught my attention and I decided to explore them.

Unforgiveness. Psychology professor and researcher Everett Worthington, Jr., instantly expanded my understanding of forgiveness by introducing me to the word *unforgiveness,* which he describes as a "jumble of emotions," including "resentment, hostility, hatred, bitterness, simmering anger and low-level fear." He goes on to say, "*Fear and anger, immediate responses, are not unforgiveness.* Unforgiveness must ripen through rumination … it takes time and reflection to develop unforgiveness." Comparing the jumbled feelings of unforgiveness to "a hot potato," Worthington acknowledges the discomfort we all feel in this state and our desire to "unload it" as soon as we can. This discomfort may lead us into forgiving too soon. Our efforts to relieve ourselves of this emotional burden include several strategies: "forbearance, successful revenge, seeing justice done, giving up the right to judge, telling a different story, and accepting the transgression."[7] Some of these strategies are born of denial and some of them are healthy coping techniques. However, only the complete process of forgiveness, which includes embracing our feelings rather than rapidly unloading them, will lead us to deep healing.

Forgiving God. Worthington's insights were in the forefront of my mind when Mary Kay revealed her feelings of unforgiveness toward God. She is furious at God because of her mother's Alzheimer's. She harbors feelings of anger and bitterness, and has completely lost her faith. Marie was a lifelong, devout Catholic, and according to Mary Kay, her mother, like Job, is completely innocent. She does *not* deserve this horrible illness in the first place, and having it linger for this length of time is unacceptable—unforgivable. As revenge, Mary Kay has disconnected from any sense of spirituality.

For more than fifteen years, Marie has lived in the nursing home. She was Mom's next-door neighbor there, so I know Marie well. She doesn't walk or talk. She can't stand or move her legs, but she can move her arms a little. I've seen her take a tissue and try to wipe her runny nose. This seemingly small effort at self-care was a large accomplishment for Marie, and quite touching and endearing to those observing this with their hearts. Marie does make some sounds, and she eats well, especially when her daughters patiently feed her. It's hard for Marie to hold up her head, so mostly she is lying in her bed or sitting slumped in her wheelchair looking at the floor. "This is not living," laments Mary Kay.

Feelings of unforgiveness toward God because of Alzheimer's are not an isolated experience happening in Mary Kay's heart alone. Surely, there are millions of people of faith who don't understand why the all-powerful God many of us learned to believe in as children allows so much suffering. Not understanding can implode into helplessness and subsequent rage when suffering enters our own lives, as it does with Alzheimer's. We are powerless to stop the losses, the decline, the financial burdens, the difficult choices, and the emotional and physical challenges.

In the circumstance of Alzheimer's, we have no place for blame, if not God. Unlike diseases caused by smoking, for example, where we can point to tobacco companies and blame them for our pain, there is no identified cause for Alzheimer's. We can't even blame the sick person who chose to smoke for exercising his or her free will in reckless ways. We don't know what to do, or not do, in order to avoid Alzheimer's. This not knowing leads many to point at God and rant.

Certain theologians look at suffering, such as Alzheimer's, and conclude that God is compassionate but has limited power and is, therefore, not responsible for causing disease. Accepting this perspective would require a complete theological overhaul for many people of faith. Some caregivers, therefore, might find more comfort in Jon Levinson's conclusions. A modern Jewish theologian, Levinson directs our attention to the varied ways that God is still "engaged in combat against powerful forces of chaos and evil in the world." Looking through the lens of the Hebrew Bible, he concludes that the vastness of God's omnipotence "has not yet fully manifested itself."[8] This interpretation holds possibility for God's current and future intervention.

Clearly, God is currently in combat with the powerful force of chaos that is Alzheimer's disease. Armies of physicians, researchers, caregivers, family members, creative and talented advocates, authors, news reporters, and even politicians have been deployed to active duty by internal calls for compassion, care, healing, and love. In the present, however, God's army is not saving Mary Kay's mom. In the cauldron of unforgiveness for this injustice, she can't forgive God and she suffers. Not surprisingly, what Mary Kay ultimately discovered as she continued to focus on caring for Marie and forgiving herself for not being able to do more was an opening that allowed the grace of God's future interventions to emerge into her heart.

Forgiving Ourselves. For two years, Mom and Marie lived next door to each other at the nursing home. Before Mary Kay and I officially met, she had seen me in Mom's room. Wheeling Marie down the hall, her first glimpse was of me washing Mom's feet. Mom had an ingrown toenail that was infected, and the foot doctor had prescribed warm water soaks in Epsom salts twice a day. Knowing that this was an added task and might overburden the aides, I did this care myself. When Mary Kay saw me, I was sitting on the floor in front of my barefooted Mom in her wheelchair. While one foot soaked, I massaged the other. During this treatment, Mom was in heaven—I could see this in her eyes. I was relaxed and grateful for the opportunity to do something tangible to help her. Partly because of Mary Kay's negative impressions of older people's feet, she perceived my foot-washing as an extraordinary act of caregiving. Over time, Mary Kay observed that I was a daily presence in Mom's life. She admired my commitment, but comparing her caregiving to mine, she feels especially inadequate in the foot washing and time spent with mom categories. Although she clearly states, "It's just too hard to see Mom like that," Mary Kay judges herself so harshly for not being emotionally stronger so she could visit daily, as she did when Marie was in the earlier stages of the disease. However, Marie has the Cadillac of wheelchairs, researched and ordered by Mary Kay. And every Sunday morning, without fail, she and her sister wash and style their mother's hair. Mary Kay's jumble of emotions is caused by love. She loves her mother so much and wants to do more for her.

As we became friends, Mary Kay shared more about her feelings of distress about Marie's illness and her unforgiveness toward herself. "I know that not going is selfish," she says. "Not going doesn't benefit Mom in anyway. It benefits me." She pauses thoughtfully after making this statement, and then adds, "Only in the short term does it benefit me not to go. But I know I'll feel guilty for the rest of my life because I didn't spend more time with her." Hoping to plant seeds of self-acceptance and self-forgiveness that would sprout within her, I consistently acknowledged Mary Kay's struggle and reminded her that she was truly doing her best under difficult circumstances.

Mary Kay really *is* doing her best as a caregiver for her mother, and she deserves forgiveness. This I know because she is earnestly engaged in both external and internal struggle. For her mother's benefit, and for her own, Mary Kay continues to challenge her emotional limits. She seeks out information and strength from others by courageously sharing her feelings. She is recognizing that small expressions of compassion—hugging her mother, scratching her back—can relieve their suffering and heal them both. Mary Kay told me about a quiet, gentle time with her mom when she scratched her back and they listened to music together, and I could feel Mary Kay transcending her pain in the holiness of those moments.

The realization that one moment of connection with her mother *does* make a difference beckons Mary Kay to step out of her own suffering and toward her mother's bedside. This, I believe, is a shining example of God's power in combat with the chaos of Alzheimer's disease—manifesting itself in and through Mary Kay. In the glow of light from the holy moments, Mary Kay tells me that she feels strong, proud, and forgiven.

Through the conventional lens of conquering disease, it does appear that God is failing in the battle against Alzheimer's. However, imagining Mary Kay and Marie basking in the light of connection and comfort, of suffering alleviated through love, what I see is a clear victory for God.

Healing Wounds from the Past. Mom was seventy-five the first time she told me how angry she was at her mother for abandoning her when she was sixteen. I was astounded by this emotional revelation at what seemed to be a late date. She had told me many times about Grandmother Philomena dying during routine gall bladder surgery as a result of physician error, but her anger was always directed toward the surgeon, toward all doctors by association. When Mom revealed her anger about being abandoned, I validated her and tried to engage her in a conversation about her feelings. Quickly, she employed a coping strategy and minimized the loss. A few years later, she brought it up again. And again, I invited her to talk about it. She didn't minimize it this time; she just didn't say more. Perhaps it was too painful for her.

Possibly Mom's anger over this abandonment festered within her soul, and she carried this heavy baggage into the world of Alzheimer's as she continued on her life journey. She may, however, have forgotten her anger. Or maybe what I hoped for actually happened. During her last years with advancing Alzheimer's, Mom had regressed to an infancy-like state, and I hoped she thought I was her mother. Social worker Naomi Feil says that a "mother's hug creates warm, safe feelings," and that a mother's face becomes recorded indelibly in the infant's brain.[9] Every day, Mom saw my loving face and received my warm hugs. I hoped that her feelings of loss and anger were replaced by the comforting awareness of being loved and safe. I hoped that, in her soul, she knew she was not abandoned and that, within her heart, the pain she felt because of her mother's death was finally healed.

Forgiving Each Other. Being human, we all hurt each other, often unintentionally. Authors Robert Browning and Roy Reed observe that we "repeatedly fail to treat each other as sacred, and instead tend to use one another in order to deal with our anxieties.[10]" It was important for my healing process to acknowledge that I had also hurt Mom in countless ways. Many of the choices I considered healing and life-affirming for me had disappointed and threatened her. In my thirties, I sent her justifiably angry letters, the kind that therapists working with abuse victims and survivors suggest we write as catharsis—but don't actually mail. I know the pain these letters caused her was searing. So it's likely that Mom also felt the jumbled emotions of unforgiveness toward me. This could explain her frequent angry outbursts and her passive-aggressive behavior toward me throughout much of my adult life.

Standing at the doorsill with Mom during the early stages of Alzheimer's, how I wished I had been able to ask her for forgiveness earlier in my life. When we began this journey together, I believed that receiving forgiveness from her would be impossible. Somewhere at the beginning of her journey, however, Mom must have forgotten her resentments toward me, since our unfolding and evolving relationship felt unburdened by my past failings. The damage to Mom's rational thinking somehow freed her and allowed her to engage and communicate with me differently. The bond between us was deepening based on the ways we validated each other in the present.

During those early years of the disease, something was happening that didn't take root in my consciousness at the time. Although neither of us had apologized, Mom must have forgiven me and instinctively moved on to the next step, which therapist Terry Hargrave refers to as "rebirthing" a relationship.[11] Through her actions, her remaining words, and her heart-speech, Mom was planting seeds for reconciliation. Although it's possible to feel forgiveness (an internal process) without engaging the person who caused the injury and without an apology from him or her, it takes two for the embrace of reconciliation (an external process) to occur.[12] In spite of her cognitive limitations, Mom reached out to me. She was initiating the embrace. I wasn't consciously aware of this until I re-read her teeny last letters almost a year after she died.

Forgiving Abusers. During the process of healing from childhood sexual abuse, which began in earnest when I was thirty-four, I experienced lingering, and sometimes overwhelming feelings of unforgiveness toward Mom—including justifiable feelings of anger and resentment—because she had not protected me from my father's abuse and because she had abandoned me, seemingly for life, through alcohol use and denial. I was therefore so surprised to spontaneously feel forgiveness for Mom in 2008 at what I thought was her deathbed. In reality, there was nothing spontaneous—that is without effort—about it. For more than twenty years, I had been actively, although unwittingly, suffering and struggling to attain forgiveness. Professor Robert D. Enright considers forgiveness "a moral choice based in struggle and suffering," which he situates biblically in his comparison of the forgiveness process to a "Refiner's Fire."[13] That April morning, when I recognized the feeling of forgiveness alive in my heart, I said "yes." Finally those burdensome feelings of unforgiveness were completely burned away. What was left was pure gold. I felt lighter. I felt kinder. I felt healed.

If forgiveness of an abuser becomes part of the healing process, according to sexual abuse conselors Ellen Bass and Laura Davis, it happens at the end of the process, only after the survivor has "gone through all the stages of remembering, grief, anger, and moving on."[14] Early in my healing, I had been warned that forgiving, and especially forgetting, wounds caused by an unrepentant abuser could be dangerous, and that *trying* to forgive could result in a "futile short circuit" of the process. Stressing the importance of safety for victims, the work of Janet Ramsey helped me understand what forgiveness is and is not, and how to protect myself.[15] Safety and trust were qualities I needed and sought in relationships. Sadly, I hadn't felt either with Mom for most of my life.

Concentrating on my own healing, I focused necessary attention on forgiving myself. Schimmel explains that sometimes people feel guilt-ridden and ashamed, harboring an inward anger that manifests as depression, even though there is no moral or rational reason for feeling this way.[16] Abused children are at particular risk for this dynamic. I had learned from abuse counselors that self-forgiveness is what's most important for healing.[17] When I began to feel forgiveness for myself for my own human failings, it just naturally extended itself to other people in the world. I started to understand humanity's limits and longings. I became able to see when somebody was doing something "right." During those early years of Alzheimer's, Mom was doing something very right, something very relational. And I was able to relationally respond to her humane, loving actions.

From remnants of my Christian upbringing, I had concluded that forgiveness was not a cognitive, willful process. In the Christian context, one can take concrete steps toward forgiveness; however, the actual experience of feeling forgiveness is a grace-filled process, "a gift from God, and a sign that God is present with us." Ramsey highlighted, for my consideration, the "impossibility of forgiveness," concluding that to forgive "is not a human achievement." She talked about some highly unlikely situations where severely injured people manage to forgive—extramarital affairs, for example. "But people do it," she said, showing the "openness for Spirit to enter the human experience. God creates the condition. We have to choose—and take radical responsibility for what we do in this world."[18]

The process for healing from abuse and the processes for experiencing forgiveness and reconciliation are similar. They all include a "deep remembering" of the wound and acknowledging feelings, including hurt, anger, hate, and shame. The processes for forgiveness and reconciliation add steps that take the abuser into consideration, inviting the wounded person to seek to understand who the abuser is, and to see if empathy is possible.[19]

Through hearing Mom describe the pain she felt over losing her driver's license and her autonomy, experiencing her losses—the labored writing on the teeny stationary, for example, noting her growing dependency and confusion, and witnessing her proud efforts to stay engaged in life and to stay in relationship with me, I recognized her vulnerability. In my own therapy, I had explored what it was like for me as a vulnerable child, helpless and afraid, with no one to protect me. And I could empathize with Mom's experience of being powerless in the presence of Alzheimer's.

"To understand everything is to forgive everything," said the Buddha. This guidance supports the modern theorists, such as Everett Worthington, who believe the key for opening the heart to forgiveness and reconciliation is empathy.[20] Each person sincerely attempts to understand the other's experience and perspective. There were things I came to understand that helped to deepen my forgiveness of Mom. For example, throughout my adult life, I learned by painful experience that trying to get persons intent on being abusive to stop is practically impossible. Maybe Mom had tried to stop my father and failed, just as I had failed to stop abusers. Maybe she had tried to protect me, but times were different then. A year before I moved to Iowa, I learned that relatives had been aware of my father's abuse. Although they took precautions to protect their own children, they didn't help Mom protect me. She was alone in an abusive situation, probably doing what she could to survive, possibly drinking to drown the pain she felt for not protecting me.

Reconciliation. A key element for reconciliation to occur is commitment. Each person refuses to give up on the other, no matter how long and difficult the process may be. Mom and I never gave up on each other.

What seemed like a miraculous event, my spontaneous forgiveness of Mom, was actually the convergence of my healing process and our unintentional steps toward reconciliation. For more than five years, through the progression of her illness, we had been creating a hopeful future for our relationship that was comprised of trust and peace.

For me, this creating process involved remembering and reflecting on Mom's helpful presence as well as the wounds she inflicted. In many ways, Mom had not protected me and she had not met my needs, but in some important ways she had done both. For example, she had been especially supportive after my two broken engagements. The first time, when I was twenty-two, she comforted me with wine and cigarettes. This showed her intention to ease my pain, although her valiant effort wasn't especially helpful. (I got very sick.) It was, however, what she knew how to do at the time. After the second broken engagement, which happened when I was fifty, I didn't even tell Mom until two months after the fact. I feared she would criticize and blame me, according to the pattern that had been established after I separated from her and her alcoholic lifestyle. Instead, hearing that I would lose my home along with my relationship, Mom surprised me by inviting me to move in with her. Although this breakup happened as Alzheimer's was beginning to manifest in Mom's brain, she was still able to express concern for my financial and physical well-being. Even more remarkable were her expressions of concern and empathy. Mom met my heartache with compassion and told me about the pain she had experienced when she was abandoned by her true love sixty years earlier. I didn't know this about Mom, and in this moment, our hearts embraced in mutual understanding.

My relationship loss became legally complicated due to jointly owned property and contractual agreements. Unfortunately, it dragged on through the court system for several years. Even though Mom's cognitive abilities kept declining during this time, she continuously showed a sincere interest in and sensitivity about my struggle. I had never before received this kind of attention from her. As her thinking weakened, it seemed as if her feelings were becoming stronger, as was her attentiveness to others and to details of personal interactions.

Immersed in the devastating aftermath of my broken relationship, my mind wasn't registering Mom's support as an indication that she had forgiven me; nor was I cognitively recognizing her extended hand as a gesture of reconciliation. My heart, however, must have been receiving her messages—loud and clear. I realize this now, because when the time came for me to meet Mom's needs, to take radical responsibility for my actions in the world, and to decide what to do when she was abandoned and alone in a nursing home, I chose our relationship —with my whole mind, heart, and soul.

Throughout the seven years between Mom's diagnosis and my decision to move to Iowa, we had been co-creating a powerfully developed sense of affiliation with each other. We had actually been rebirthing a lasting, trusting relationship. Although I was not being deliberate and was not conscious of my intentions —and I assume Mom wasn't either, we had been living out what Browning and Reed identify as our "basic human desire for attachment,"[21] a desire apparently not deterred by Alzheimer's disease.

According to Professor Earl Thompson, the process of reconciliation is more than dialogue; it necessarily includes action. He continues, "For true reconciliation to occur, the people *must* be changed. They *must* break with the past and move toward a new future of amendment and restitution." [22] Mom and I were both changed by my healing and by her Alzheimer's. Her past was gone, forgotten. I haven't cognitively forgotten the ways Mom wounded me in the past, and if necessary or useful, I can tell the story in detail; however, my life-long painful feelings of abandonment and betrayal *are* forgotten. My feelings of hurt and anger have been displaced, and I'm now surrounded by warm feelings of being loved, accepted, and taken care of by my mom. The feeling of being safe in the arms of a loving, protective mother—forever—is what I hoped I could give to her, how I hoped I would help heal her soul from the wounds of a lifetime of abandonment. Surprisingly, this is exactly what she gave to me. This is how she healed me.

Mom's and my openness to forgiveness and our actions toward reconciliation miraculously triumphed over extreme familial abuse and Alzheimer's disease. Martin Buber explains how this can happen: "In the beginning is the relation."[23] Mom recognized our relationship and she reached out. I reached back, discovering that in the beginning, at the end, and during every precious moment in between—longing, loving, living, being, and truly meeting each other, who we were, where we were, how we were—it was all about relationship.

Nourishing Compassion

We need one another. There is no question about this. On the journey of life, we *always* need one another—but at certain times, this need is more apparent than at others. Writer George Odell recognizes some of these certain times:

> We need one another when we mourn and would be comforted.
>
> We need one another when we are in trouble and afraid.
>
> We need one another when we are in despair, in temptation, and need to be recalled to our best selves again.
>
> We need one another when we would accomplish some great purpose, and cannot do it alone.
>
> We need one another in the hour of success, when we look for someone to share our triumphs.
>
> We need one another in the hour of defeat, when with encouragement we might endure, and stand again.
>
> We need one another when we come to die, and would have gentle hands prepare us for the journey.
>
> All our lives we are in need, and others are in need of us.[24]

We are an interdependent species, more radically dependent on love than any other beings. Scholar Karen Armstrong explains, "Our brains have evolved to be caring and to need care—to such an extent that they are impaired if this nurture is lacking."[25] The end of life is a particularly vulnerable time and those who are leaving us need our greatest compassion.

One of the challenging realities we meet when our loved ones are diagnosed with Alzheimer's is that the length of time we spend preparing them for the journey to the other side of this illness could be quite long. Although Alzheimer's is a terminal disease, it is not a sentence of imminent death. Acknowledging this, some researchers and caregivers have described Alzheimer's disease as death in slow motion. David Shenk explains it eloquently:

> As the disease relentlessly progresses toward the final dimming of the sufferer, it forces us to experience death in a way that is rarely otherwise experienced. What is usually a quick flicker, we see in super slow motion, over years. It is more painful than many people can even imagine, but it is also perhaps the most poignant of all reminders of why and how human life is so extraordinary. It is our best lens on the meaning of loss.[26]

This chronic disease of progressive losses reveals what it means to live and love to our fullest potential, including our potential for compassion.

People with Alzheimer's are continually changing, continually dying, as we all are. As I so exquisitely learned, however, they aren't gone until they have taken their last breaths. From within their long walks toward death, persons with Alzheimer's continually extend invitations to us to practice compassion and kindness, and to love them through all the changes of their lives.

I witnessed this invitation every day as I walked down the hall-way of the nursing home. When persons with dementia saw me, they extended their hands and pleaded for connection—for a touch, a hug, a glass of water. Many simply pleaded, "Help me."

From the beginning of my journey through Alzheimer's with Mom, I experienced the reaching and pleading of those afflicted with this disease as an opportunity to broaden my world view in order to make a place in my heart and in my life for "the other," which Armstrong identifies as an impor-tant attitude for fostering compassion.[27] Observing the care provided to residents by some of the nursing home staff, I wit-nessed, with awe, the many ways they manifested compassion as Armstrong defines and describes it: "Compassion impels us to work tirelessly to alleviate the suffering of our fellow creatures, to dethrone ourselves from the centre of our world and put another there, and to honour the inviolable sanctity of every single human being, treating everybody, without exception, with absolute justice, equity, and respect."[28]

Anyone who has spent time in nursing homes observing aides and nurses caring for the residents, particularly residents who are completely helpless, will readily be able to distinguish between the caring professionals Sam Keen refers to as "care-sellers"[29] and those who are working tirelessly to alleviate suf-fering and honor the sanctity of every person. Although I don't harshly judge the care-sellers—everyone has to work for a living —they give only the services they are paid to give. They have learned how to implement tasks from their rational being, as noted by bioethicist Jeffrey Bishop. The compassionate caring that Armstrong describes is given for free, from the heart. Bishop claims that care is an action originating in the bodies and souls of the caregivers. Care requires this intention to be directed, by our bodies and our souls, at the bodies and souls of those who need care. Caregivers are called to take away pain, not with pills but with the offering of self.[30]

When the nursing home policy evolved, allowing me to choose Mom's primary care aides, I chose Julie to care for Mom during the morning shift, which began at 5:30 AM. This remains one of my life's best choices. Julie had been working with the elderly for her whole career—over thirty years—because she cared. I saw that Julie's caring for my mother (and all her residents) was what Bishop calls a "fully embodied activity" that came from "desire."[31]

The most important gift any of us can receive at times of loss, pain, or need is steadfast presence. "Caring is messy," says Bishop, "and inefficient."[32] End-of-life incontinence, believe me, is messy. And because this mess requires immediate attention, it undermines a caregiver's efficiency. No matter how big the mess, however, Julie never retreated from my mom. She was there six mornings a week, before many of us were even out of bed, attending to Mom's needs—whatever they were.

Although Julie's full-time schedule required her to work five days a week, she regularly volunteered to work an additional day. She understood how important consistency was to her residents, all of whom had Alzheimer's or some other form of dementia. This consistency of compassionate, patient, quality care—demonstrated by Julie's commitment and attachment to her residents—was part of what made Mom's nursing home experience and Julie's work successful. Personal attachment to residents, according to Bishop, is the key element that prevents burnout.[33] Instead of dreading coming to work, resisting the physical demands, and avoiding the incontinence messes, Julie volunteered for more of this.

Compassion should not be confused with pity, states Armstrong. It's not about feeling sorry for those in need.[34] "True compassion," according to Buddhist teacher Pema Chödrön, "does not come from wanting to help out those less fortunate than ourselves, but from realizing one's kinship with all beings."[35] Other spiritual teachers echo this definition. Armstrong writes,

"Compassion means to endure with another person, to put ourselves in someone else's shoes, to feel her pain as though it were our own, and to enter generously into his point of view."[36] Richard Rohr says, "Love is recognizing oneself in the other."[37] Jesus scholar Marcus Borg adds the element of being inspired by the feeling into action: "Compassion thus means feeling the feelings of somebody else in a visceral way, at a level somewhere below the level of the head; most commonly associated with feeling the suffering of somebody else and being moved by that suffering to do something. That is, the feeling of compassion leads to being compassionate."[38]

Julie may not have allowed herself to personally identify with the complete vulnerability of her residents. She told me, however, that she did identify them with her own mother, who had suffered and died years earlier. Julie had dearly cared for her as well. Many of the aides and nurses who were freely giving compassionate care echoed Julie's experience of caring for the residents as if they were "their own." Borg tells his readers that, in the Hebrew language, the singular form of *compassion* is translated as "womb." Being compassionate, therefore, "has nuances of giving life, nourishing, caring, perhaps embracing and encompassing."[39]

Both Bishop and Rohr speak about the connection between care and relationship. According to Bishop, babies *require* warm caring and friendliness in order for them to survive.[40] In his discussion of the "True and False Self," Rohr acknowledges that we are social creatures. In order to be truly loved, we need to be vulnerable with another and allow ourselves to be seen in our "littleness." "Someone else," Rohr says, has to see our vulnerability and "acknowledge us as beloved."[41]

This was Julie's specialty. Her skills of observation were acute—she saw Mom's vulnerability, which Mom and all the residents had no choice but to reveal. She listened well to my description of Mom's needs and desires, and fulfilled them with joy. And she helped Mom to feel good about herself. During the last two years of Mom's life, when Julie accompanied her to the bathroom for toileting, washing, and tooth-brushing, Julie sang to her the 1974 hit song "You Are So Beautiful to Me."

Imagine beginning every morning with someone singing, "You're everything I hoped for. . . . Such joy and happiness you bring,"[42] and feeling that you are beloved on this earth. After singing to Mom, Julie dressed her in a coordinated outfit, brushed her long hair and spritzed it with water to bring out the natural waves, decorated her hair with colorful or flowered clips, and then chose a necklace to complete her ensemble. Six days out of seven, when I arrived to spend time with Mom, she had already been awakened and cared for by a person who was the embodiment of compassion. Witnessing this care, appreciating this care, I concluded that Julie was another of Mom's soul mates, compassionately guiding her home.[43]

Julie was also part of our carepartnering circle. Her care extended beyond Mom to me. Because she had cared for her own sick and dying mother, Julie could identify with my fears, worries, and struggles. She knew that Mom's quality of life and well-being were important to me, and made extra effort to ensure that my needs and wants for Mom's care, as specified in the care plan, were met. What Julie received from me—which Mom couldn't give her—were regular expressions of gratitude for her attention to details and her gentle kindness. While Julie was singing, Mom did tend to look at her through starry eyes, so Julie knew Mom appreciated her. But hearing "thank you" every day from families and knowing that their efforts are noticed, gives nursing aides an energy boost. Being appreciated gives everyone a boost.

Julie wasn't working the morning Mom died. As soon as Mom was gone, however, a close coworker called her, knowing that Jeanne's life and death mattered to her. Julie dropped what she was doing when she got the call and came immediately to the nursing home to be at Mom's bedside and say good-bye. She also came to comfort and share her grief with me. She felt the loss of her friend and companion Jeanne. Julie was grateful that she wasn't working that day, so she was able to experience the fullness of her grief without needing to attend to other residents.

This experience of loss is the challenge for compassionate health care workers in nursing homes who become personally attached to those destined to die soon. Their job is to get people ready to die. Person after person after person, these compassionate carers must say goodbye to their friends and feel the loss when they leave.

Julie sat beside me at Mom's funeral and held my hand.

As I've talked with other family members who have loved ones with dementia and other diminishments living in nursing homes, some have said, "I don't visit Dad (Mom, my brother, my sister, my aunt, my uncle, etc.) at the nursing home (or hospital) because he wouldn't want anyone to see him like that."

I wonder if this is really true. Diminishment is indeed hard to experience and hard to witness, but if we put aside our vanity and egotism, is that what people really want? Is that what *we* want— for our imperfect humanity, our "littleness"—to be invisible to those we love? As writer Mary Vineyard says, "It takes radical and radiant humility to accept our helplessness and bow to the necessity of being cared for by family members and strangers."[44]

In the humbleness of my humanity, I know it would be painful for me to be sick, confused, vulnerable, unable to speak or walk, and left alone in a nursing home, helpless to fend for myself. Because it would be devastatingly painful for me to be abandoned at my time of greatest need, I chose not to inflict this pain on my mother.

At the time, I wasn't consciously aware that my choice to protect Mom from abandonment was a reflection of the Golden

Rule: Do unto others as you would have them do unto you. As originally taught by Confucius in China over twenty-five hundred years ago, the Golden Rule invites us to "look into our own hearts, discover what gives us pain, and then refuse, under any circumstance whatsoever, to inflict this pain on anybody else." About a hundred years later in India, the Buddha introduced a practice of meditation on the "four elements of the 'immeasurable' love that exists within everything." The Buddhist tradition describes compassion, one of these four elements, as the determination to free those who are suffering from their pain. These early traditions agree that compassion is not only natural to humans but what Armstrong calls "the fulfillment of human nature."[45]

Around 300 BCE, the Confucian philosopher Mencius was the first to challenge humanity to cultivate what he called our natural "shoots" of compassion, claiming that once cultivated, our compassion will then acquire a "dynamic power of its own." According to Armstrong, human beings have always been prepared to work hard to enhance a natural ability. Consider the evolution from the self-protective running and jumping skills of our ancestors to the graceful physical abilities of ballet dancers or gymnasts that result from years of dedicated practice. This demonstrates the irrefutable reality that, if we persevere, we can acquire an ability that at first seemed impossible. "In this same way," Armstrong says, "those who have persistently trained themselves in the art of compassion manifest new capacities in the human heart and mind; they discover that when they reach out consistently toward others, they are able to live with the suffering that inevitably comes their way with serenity, kindness and creativity."[46]

Ancient sages, prophets, and mystics from all religious traditions did not regard compassion as an impossible dream. They worked as hard to implement compassion in the difficult circumstances of their lives as our social structure works today to identify the cause of and find a cure for Alzheimer's disease. Although Armstrong believes that compassion is intrinsic in all human beings, she also believes that each of us needs to work diligently to cultivate and expand our capacity for compassion.

I've become convinced that this disease of relentless diminishment has come, seemingly as a scourge upon our world, to remind us that the well of compassion will never run dry, and that, in fact, the more we draw on it the more we have. Taking our inspiration from the ancient sages, we caregivers need to remind society that nourishing our shoots of compassion as earnestly as science searches for cures is an important manifestation of our humanity. According to Borg, this reminder to society would be a faith-filled response, since this was also the work of Jesus. "For Jesus," Borg writes, "compassion was more than a quality of God and an individual virtue: it was a social paradigm, the core value for life in community."[47]

Almost eighteen months after Mom died, I attended the Joy of Caring Conference, where I met Dr. Bishop. During one of his presentations, he introduced participants to an icon from the Greek Orthodox tradition, the *Dormition of the Theokotos* ("The Falling Asleep of the Holy Mother of God").[48] In this stunning painting depicting Mary's death, Jesus stands behind her human body holding a baby, which represents Mary's soul. Because icons present an experience artistically through pictures rather than words, they are emotionally evocative. Just as one of the contemplative spiritual practices recommended by St. Ignatius of Loyola encourages us to place ourselves in the Gospels as we read them,[49] I placed myself into this icon. In my imagination, it was I who was given the blessed opportunity to tenderly hold my mother's spirit, in the form of an infant, during those last years when Alzheimer's was in the late and end stages.

This tender holding of Mom's body and soul in my hands over several years was cultivating my compassion, even if I

269

didn't fully realize it at the time. Almost two years after Mom died, an encounter at the nursing home made me aware of how much my compassion had grown. I had not been back there since cleaning out Mom's belongings from her room and saying good-bye to the staff. Although many family members do return as volunteers after their loved ones die, I couldn't bring myself to return. Then a friend had knee-replacement surgery. After leaving the hospital, he was transferred to Mom's nursing home for rehabilitation. I seized the moment and went one morning to join him for Mass and then to see about helping with the exercise class Mom and I had loved. As I stepped into the elevator on my way to the chapel, I saw a resident in her wheelchair. She was leaning over the side of her chair, drooling. She was still wearing her pajamas, which had remnants of breakfast smeared down the front. Her hands were nervously rubbing the arms of her chair, and she was making sounds as she looked with pleading eyes at the man running the elevator. This was a remarkable moment for me. Earlier in my life, I would have felt disgust, horror, judgment, or fear while observing this woman; perhaps I would have fled from the nursing home the instant the elevator door opened. On this day, however, after years of nourishing my "shoots" by caring for Mom, the only feeling I noticed was the compassion for this woman that was overflowing in my heart. This feeling nudged me to take compassionate action. I have returned to the nursing home as a volunteer, helping to lead the exercise class. Apparently, I make it fun for the residents. At least this is what Katrina, one of the exercisers, told me.

Very recently, I noticed another change in my capacity for compassion. I was walking in the late afternoon as I usually do, and I unexpectedly re-remembered a childhood experience that I have always considered to be one of Mom's terrible parenting moments.

It was a Saturday evening in the summer when I was five.

My parents were getting ready to go out for the night to play bridge with their friends. This every-other-Saturday night ritual was the extent of their social life. I had gone to the store with some neighbors to buy candy. As we walked home through an alley shortcut, I stumbled on the loose gravel, falling and cutting my leg on a piece of glass. It was a long, deep cut. Blood gushed from the wound and I was hysterical. When the neighbors brought me home to Mom, she was furious. Dad quickly exited from the bloody, emotional scene and went to pick up the babysitter. Mom sat me on a wooden chair in her bedroom and hurriedly tried to clean and bandage the cut as I screamed and sobbed and squirmed. Mom's voice was harsh; her handling of my wounded leg was rough; her facial expression was mean. Somehow the bandaging was accomplished, the babysitter arrived, and my parents went out to play cards.

Mom must have harbored vivid memories of this night as well, and presumably she felt guilty about it. For years and years after the event, she brought my attention to the three-inch long scar on my left leg, saying she should have taken me to the hospital for stitches. It was this scar, and this scar alone, she said, that would prevent me from being Miss America. Hearing this, my fragile self-esteem was maimed.

Historically, in my memory of this story, there was cruelty layered upon cruelty. I interpreted Mom's behavior to mean that playing cards was more important than caring for and comforting her injured and terrified child. But as I re-remembered this story with enhanced compassion, I could see it from different perspectives. I saw my Mom's life as wife and mother in the 1950s. The era and these roles were limiting for creative, enterprising women, stifling and depressing for many. Since she accepted her expected roles of wife and mother reluctantly, Mom didn't have an especially happy marriage or fulfilling life.

It was their one night out. Mom's one night in fourteen away from the demands of children and housewifely duties. This night out was important to my parents. They hired a babysitter and took time and effort to get ready. Dad wore a suit and tie. Mom wore a fancy dress, nylon hose, high heels, and a necklace with matching clip-on earrings. She was looking forward to being free from responsibility and having fun with friends when her clumsy, crying child threatened to spoil her reprieve.

With my enhanced compassion, this story became more expansive for me. It's larger now than the pain, fear, and hurt feelings I experienced. In the context of Mom's unhappy life, she didn't see me fully. Overwhelmed by the prospect of disappointment or concerned about the cost of a visit to the emergency room, Mom didn't realize how her words and actions would wound me.

Through most of my life, Mom didn't see me. However, my increasing capacity for compassion, which developed over my years of caring for her, helped me to see her—and to continue seeing her even after her death.

I now see how and why caring for Mom was, indeed, an especially good fortune in my life. There is perhaps no greater gift than the opportunity to alleviate another human being's suffering through compassionate caring.

After all my years of observing and studying about Alzheimer's disease, I've concluded that we really need the ones who are slowly declining from this and other diseases of dementia. Dying people have a purpose beyond showing us how to fight to conquer every disease. They are giving us countless opportunities to acknowledge and enhance our natural human tendencies toward compassion, and to practice being loving and kind and patient. They are encouraging us, needing us, to nourish our innate compassion into its full dynamic power.

Author Martha Beck points out that, when frightened, all mammals except humans will seek a safe place, but humans seek a safe person.[50] I was Mom's safe person during her time of need. Compassion had made it possible.

Redefining Survival

O ver the past sixteen years, more than twenty thousand families, mine included, have sought support from the Alzheimer's Association office in Dubuque, Iowa. Considering the geographic location, which includes one small city and surrounding rural areas, this number is stunning. Even more stunning is that only a handful of people helped by the association have returned there as volunteers. Dubuque's annual Walk to End Alzheimer's attracts a small percentage of the people touched by the diseases of dementia, past and present. Compared to the numbers of walkers and contributions received through similar fundraising programs, such as for breast cancer, diabetes, or heart disease, the Alzheimer's effort has miniscule support.

It's the same all across the country: fewer volunteers, walkers, and rally participants and less financial support. Hearing this sparked my curiosity. "Why is this the case?" I asked the Alzheimer's Association staff member who shared this news with me. She answered without hesitation: "Because there are no survivors."

This reality, so bluntly stated, gave me pause. Although I had gone to the Association's office to talk about volunteering and leading programs for other caregivers, the prospect of no survivors made me want to run away and never return. My heart cried out, "It's so true!" Alzheimer's, like life, leaves no survivors. Accordingly, there are no victory celebrations honoring those who have fought the good fight against Alzheimer's disease and won.

For a brief time following this conversation, the idea of no survivors—which I accepted as the truth of Alzheimer's—seized my heart, seemingly choking my open-heartedness toward this population. It guided me away from the disease and the diminishments, and I got lost. Eventually, as I allowed myself to wonder more about surviving and Alzheimer's, I began to realize that my automatic reaction was a reflection of what I consider the conventional wisdom of our society. Because our primary focus is on conquering disease, the scientific, medical, and most common understanding of the word *survivor* is often used in its narrowest meaning: "one who remains alive."

Marcus Borg, through his discussion of alternative wisdom,[51] and Pema Chödrön, who encourages us to use the life we already have to make us wiser rather than more stuck,[52] encouraged my heart to beat once again in solidarity with persons with Alzheimer's and their caregivers. If we look at Alzheimer's disease through the lens of alternative wisdom, which Borg notes is often the province of philosophers and spiritual sages, not scientists,[53] the concept of survival reveals a goal more consistent with healing than with curing. Through this lens, *to survive* means "to continue to function or manage in spite of some adverse circumstance or hardship; hold up; endure." According to this definition, persons with Alzheimer's could be considered the ultimate survivors. Every single day of their long journeys, Alzheimer's survivors face loss and adversity. And every single day, for up to twenty years, they endure, adapt, function, and live to endure and adapt another day.

Their survival is marked by resiliency, compensating for losses, reconfiguring life and relationships, healing, and transforming.

When this understanding of survival is embraced by Alzheimer's caregivers, we also do more than just get through it alive. We grow, we become wiser, and we can actually thrive as we walk on, making room in our lives for all that is real. Borg describes a purpose for the wisdom we will acquire: "It speaks for the nature of reality and how to live one's life in accord with reality."[54]

As I continue to seek meaning in my life, I return to the world of Alzheimer's. I return to this world where people are authentic, where they are meeting reality with honesty and resilience, and where they are surviving every day. I return because it abounds with opportunities to make a difference, and with wisdom to help me find my own way home through this mysterious maze of my mortal life. I return to the world of Alzheimer's because connecting with people who have no hope of conquering their diseases, as well as with caregivers who are seeking ways to care for and connect with their loved ones, I feel awash in the presence of God. I recognize and feel the Spirit of Life and Love manifesting all around me as longing for connection, and manifesting within me as compassion, respect, and gratitude for those who still have much to show me about living. Through my relationship with Mom, which inspires me even after her death, I continue to make discoveries that encourage and enlighten me as I walk on.

A few months after Mom died, I attended a six-week grief support group offered by a local hospice organization. The group was a safe, helpful way to explore my feelings of loss in the company of others who respected my process. One woman in the group said that, on her husband's birthday, she and her children took helium balloons to the cemetery and released them as they sang happy birthday. What an outstanding idea! I began this ritual immediately.

On Mother's Day, on Mom's birthday, and on the anniversary of the day she died, I buy a single balloon displaying an appropriate message for the occasion and attach a small card with my thoughts about this day and my wishes for Mom on her journey. I take the balloon and card to the cemetery, release the balloon, and watch it rise and float on the air, south down the Mississippi River.

The balloon always floats south, it seems, and I solemnly watch until it's gone from my sight. I'm careful not to blink or to glance away at anything else even for a moment, so as to prolong my sensory connection to the balloon and its message for Mom. I imagine it will reach her.

On the second anniversary of Mom's death, I watched as the balloon rose high, floated far away on the wings of the wind, and then disappeared from my view. Although the small speck eventually moved out of the range of my vision, I knew with my whole being, with certainty beyond any doubt, that it was still there, still floating, still on the way to its unknown destination. In that fleeting, extraordinary instant, I felt connected to Mom in her new world, to the whole universe, and to whatever lies beyond it. At that moment, Sarah Young's interpretation of 2 Corinthians from my morning meditation returned to my consciousness: "Things that are visible are brief and fleeting, while things that are invisible are everlasting."[55]

Walking home from the cemetery, I wondered what else exists beyond my eyes' ability to see, beyond the reach of my other senses, beyond the comprehension of my mind? Savoring this expansive moment of deep encounter, I also wondered when the next unexpected glorious mystery would cross my path, and what it would be. Walking on toward healing and wholeness, I know that wherever my path leads me, presence and wonder will always be my faithful companions.

Companionship
on the Journey

As cognition declines, persons with Alzheimer's—and family caregivers as well—tend to become isolated. The reasons for this outcome are many and varied, and they include: shame about revealing diminished capacities, possible rejection by frightened family members and friends who don't know what to do or say, confusion about what's happening, frustration, fear, and pure exhaustion. Looking back at my own experiences, I realize that having companionship can be a determining factor as to whether caregiving will become a burden or a blessing.

Years ago, a friend from a twelve-step program observed what he referred to as my greatest strength: the ability to ask for and accept help. Nowhere in my life has this strength been needed or more life-giving than on my journey with Mom through Alzheimer's disease.

As professors, colleagues, and friends listened to me and read about my caregiving experiences with Mom throughout the years, they noticed that something seemed to be missing. I wasn't suffering. They didn't understand. Since other family caregivers talking about and writing about Alzheimer's often seem burdened and in great pain over the stresses and losses inherent in the disease, I didn't really understand myself. Because I wasn't suffering, I thought maybe I was doing something wrong—*until* I started making the list of my companions, teachers, and guides on this journey.

I had come to Iowa—alone—to be with Mom. Having been away from my hometown for thirty-two years, I didn't know anyone except Mom. I knew, however, that I needed help—to learn about the disease, become an effective caregiver, address my fears, find a place to live, meet compatible people, develop a support system, take care of myself, find spiritual inspiration, and make sure Mom had the best care and the best quality of life possible. So, I reached out. I asked for what I needed—and I received information, guidance, companionship, and support beyond anything I could have imagined. I didn't want Mom to suffer with this disease any more than was absolutely necessary. Surprisingly, my efforts to relieve her suffering also relieved my own suffering.

With gratitude for each and every one of my companions, teachers, and guides, I share my list as an acknowledgment of their contributions and as encouragement for all Alzheimer's caregivers to ask for what we need. Help is available . . . just waiting for us to seek, to ask, and to find.

The companions, teachers, and guides who helped me to see the Spirit of Life shining through Alzheimer's include:

authors and poets
musicians and singers
mystics and theologians—ancient and modern
professors at Andover Newton Theological School, Weston
    Jesuit School of Theology, and Boston College
healers of all kinds—counselors, spiritual directors, doctors
spiritual directors' peer groups in Massachusetts and Iowa
my centering prayer group

friends and colleagues whose parents and spouses also had/have Alzheimer's

daughters and sons at the nursing home

spouses at the nursing home

many friends—old and new friends, near and far-away friends

one very good friend at the nursing home who shared the experience with me on a daily basis for almost four years

church services

my lawyer, Werner Hellmer, a wise and trusted advisor for more than six years

Mom's doctors—Dr. Angela Kelley, the primary care physician, who could see Mom's worth and dignity; Dr. Allen Meurer, the physician who examined Mom regularly at the nursing home, who came to see her on her deathbed and cried with me; and all the doctors in the emergency room who always treated Mom with the same respect and care given to every other patient

carepartners at the nursing home—the nursing aides, especially Karen, Julie, Angela, Angelic, Roxanne, Tracey, Kim, and Dawn; the nurses; the social workers; the speech therapists; the occupational therapists; the food service staff; the administrator; the activities staff; and the advocates, especially Jan

emergency room and hospital staff

hospice staff—especially Kelly, Amy, Cindy, Stephanie, Penny, Ashley, and Harold

Alzheimer's Association staff in Iowa and Massachusetts

my newly found, dear cousin, Ron

the Sisters of St. Francis and the staff at the Shalom Retreat Center, who welcomed me to Iowa, made a home for me, and prayed with me

> the nursing home residents, especially the dear ones with
> Alzheimer's
> Mom, my most faithful, my most beloved companion

I specifically want to acknowledge and express my appreciation to the following individuals who personally guided me
and supported me throughout the journey, and who helped me
mold and fashion this book:

Sister Catherine Griffiths, my beloved spiritual guide, was the
one clear, unwavering voice encouraging me to follow my call
to care for my mother.

Lindsay Brennan and Mary McNally worked for the Alzheimer's
Association during my journey. They provided compassionate
care and patient guidance as I wandered through the mysterious, sometimes thorny maze of Alzheimer's caregiving. Lindsay
also recognized my unique vision and approach to caregiving
and wholeheartedly encouraged me to share my vision with
others, as did Melanie Chavin from the Illinois Chapter.

As I was searching for a better way to care for Mom during
the earlier stages of her illness, Joanne Koenig Coste and Dr.
William Berlingieri taught this curious, eager novice so much
about effective caregiving. Due to their previous observations, I
was able to step off the high dive into the ocean of Alzheimer's
care, feeling confident and competent. For generously sharing
their wisdom, Mom and I are forever grateful.

Learning the craft of improvisation from David La Graffe and
Will Luera transformed my life. My inspiration to transfer the
skills of improvisation into Alzheimer's caregiving also transformed Mom's life—from potential isolation to a life rich with
connection. And now, as I pass on the skills I learned from David

and Will to other caregivers, the ripples in the pool started by their gems of knowledge and joy grow larger and larger.

Even after discovering ways to connect with Mom through improvisation, I remained terrified and mostly avoidant about the hard facts of Alzheimer's disease. At a Healing Moments workshop on Cape Cod during the spring of 2008, I had the great pleasure of meeting Lisa Genova, who generously gifted me with a copy of *Still Alice*, her novel about early-onset Alzheimer's. Lisa's use of fiction to engage and enlighten readers about such a difficult subject was remarkably effective. This book gently opened my mind, giving me the courage I needed to read more and more on the subject of Alzheimer's.

Dr. Brita Gill-Austern was the midwife for this work. She and other professors in the Doctor of Ministry Program at Andover Newton Theological School, Dr. Earl Thompson and Dr. Jennifer Peace, who gave me the opportunity to creatively integrate my personal journey with my academic endeavors. What a gift this has been for my heart and my soul!

On the journey through Alzheimer's, I was blessed to encounter other family caregivers who embraced me with their open, loving hearts. Mary Anne, Coleen, Mary Kay, Carl, and Stephen agreed to explore their experiences and feelings, and share them with me for this resource for other caregivers. Their perspectives enlarged my own and helped me to see and hear, with amazement, the miracles that are around us always. Caregiver Betsy Peterson also generously shared her story with me as well as her comfortable and beautiful home.

My colleagues in the Healing Moments Alzheimer's Ministry, Rev. Laura Randall, Rev. Darrick Jackson, Amy Ressler, David La Graffe, Jill Seiler-Moon, Rev. Esther Hurlburt, and Coleen

Hein, have been my committed travelling companions. They have given my ideas wings.

My soul sisters—Robbie, Diane, Nancy, Carla Owen, Kelly, Bonnie, Janaan, Marilyn, and Cathy—encourged me through the challenging twists of this project and embraced me at every celebration. Their presence in my life has taught me much about myself and much about friendship.

Barbara Day brought expertise and graciousness to the technical editing process, and words will never express the magnitude of my appreciation for her skill.

Mary Benard, editorial director at Skinner House Books, believed in this project from the beginning. Her vision gave me direction, and her commitment encouraged me to persevere through the daunting parts of the publication process. Mary's attention to detail inspired awe, and her calm presence and consistent good cheer filled me with admiration. Mary's contributions, and every contribution to the creation of this book by the Skinner House staff—Marshall Hawkins, Betsy Martin, Kate Bates, and Joni McDonald—have been deeply appreciated. Suzanne Morgan's sensitive attention to the cover art and the design of this book are especially appreciated. The day the cover image arrived was a day of pure joy for me and for the photographer Coleen, since the woman in the photo with the butterfly on her arm is Coleen's mom and my dear friend, Ilene.

The support of the Editorial Board of Skinner House Books gave me a feeling of deep pride for the innovative and compassionate positions consistently taken by the Unitarian Universalist Association. Alzheimer's disease is a topic truly needing spiritual attention, and I'm grateful that my religious denomination has so directly taken the leadership to heal the millions of wounded souls affected by this disease. Through the Board's decision to publish this book, the UUA has once again demonstrated its commitment to stand on the side of love.

Rev. Libbie Stoddard and Gary Whited have been my mentors and guides for more than twenty years, and to them, I am most grateful. I owe much of who I now am, and what I have accomplished in my life, to them. They saw my potential and believed in me, encouraged me, and loved me during all those years when Mom couldn't. Unquestionably, their presence in my life aided my healing and made it possible for me to care for Mom when she needed me.

Although I'm sad my mom had to take the path through Alzheimer's disease on her way home, I am eternally grateful that she reached out to me during her time of need and let me know that my presence in her life was helpful and healing. It was through her decline and resulting vulnerability, and through her initiative, that our relationship was restored. I hope that the stories of Mom's courageous meeting with Alzheimer's, her willingness to humbly ask for help (something she had never had to do before), and her ability to recognize kindness will be endearing and inspiring to others. Mom would be so happy to know that, through her example, our experiences together, and my writing, she has been able to help someone else in need.

Resources for Caregivers

Reflection Questions

When did the relationship shift so that you took on the role of caregiver? Was there a defining moment?

What are some moments in your role as caregiver that have brought you joy?

What moments with your loved one with dementia have brought you a sense of fulfillment?

What have you learned about life and love?

What has been your most valuable lesson?

What has been your greatest challenge?

What has been your greatest loss?

Even as your loved one's capacities have diminished, what has made their life valuable …

    to them?
    to you?
    to society?

What has surprised you about the quality of your relationship with your loved one even as the dementia has increased?

What has surprised you most about your loved one's remaining capacities?

What aspects of her/his personality have they retained?

What has motivated you to alter your life to care for your loved one?

What have been some of the most remarkable experiences with your loved one?
Why?

How have you grown spiritually throughout the course of your loved one's illness?

Spiritual Practices

The most important aspects of any spiritual practice are making the time and following through on a commitment to do it, no matter how we feel and no matter how challenging the circumstances become. It's about showing up, with our hearts open to receiving grace, guidance, and support.

Alzheimer's caregiving provides an opportunity for spiritual practice that will ultimately benefit both the caregiver and the care-receiver. As a place to begin, I suggest that the most important spiritual endeavors for Alzheimer's caregivers are prayer and the spiritual practices of acceptance, mindfulness, and self-care.

Prayer

Over the years, as I worked on healing from my history of abuse, the Serenity Prayer[1] had become important to me. When Alzheimer's became a part of my life, I altered this prayer in ways that supported my process. I offer my altered prayer as a sample to other caregivers. Use this prayer, find one that's meaningful to you, or create your own:

God, grant me
the Serenity
> to accept the things I cannot change:
> the predictable, relentless diminishment that is
> > Alzheimer's;
> the ongoing losses;
> the mysteries embedded in this disease that
> > continue to elude explanation and cure;

the courage
> to change the things I can:
> my attitude, my reactions, my expectations, my
> > priorities;

And the wisdom to know the difference.

God, may I open my heart to the peace that passes all
understanding.
May I care for and comfort my loved one with patience
and compassion.
May I be Hope.

Amen.

Prayer for Help. Caregivers need not hesitate to pray for help. I've heard it said that the simple prayer, "Help me," is one of the truest prayers we can say. Perhaps repeating this prayer will allow caregivers to realize that needing and receiving help are necessary for sustaining life. None of us can get through this life or Alzheimer's alone.

Prayer of Gratitude. Meister Eckhart, a German Christian mystic living in the thirteenth century, wrote: "If a man had no more to do with God than to be thankful, that would suffice."[2]

Every day, even the difficult ones, it has become a powerful practice for me to notice one thing for which I feel gratitude. One thing: Today I am grateful to NOT have a headache. David Steindl-Rast says, "It's not the happy people who are grateful. It's the grateful people who are happy."[3]

Prayer for Gratitude and Acceptance. Dag Hammarskjold, a twentieth-century Swedish diplomat with a spiritual worldview, offers care partners what I consider the most healing prayer of all. The prayer includes an apt expression of feelings shared by many persons with Alzheimer's and their caregivers and goes on to address both memory and hope:

> For all that has been—Thank you!
> For all that shall be—Yes![4]

Acceptance

Research has identified acceptance as the only coping technique to significantly reduce caregiver stress and distress. It's therefore imperative to become informed about Alzheimer's disease, so you know what to accept and how. Make the time and find the courage to listen to CDs and watch DVDs, read books, attend support groups and seminars, and connect with the Alzheimer's Association and other caregivers. Understanding the disease and how it's intersecting with your loved one's personality, and knowing that your loved one is doing the best they can 100 percent of the time will ease your need and desire to control what can't be controlled or to change what can't be changed. Caregivers need not be alone on this journey. Seeking companions and accepting help could transform a potentially burdensome experience into a blessing.

Mindfulness

Pay attention to your loved one and yourself. Enhance your outer and your inner vision. Mindfulness will help you know what you need, how your loved one is doing, and what they might need or want. Persons with Alzheimer's aren't the best reporters of how they're feeling, medication side effects, whether they've had lunch, if their shoes hurt or their pants are too tight. Being able to notice and interpret sounds, facial expressions, and mood changes is a critical skill for caregivers to learn. In the early stages, when persons with Alzheimer's are aware of their diminishing capacities, they may intentionally disguise their vulnerabilities. For example, instead of acknowledging that they don't understand what you said, they may laugh or respond in a way that seems appropriate. Mom had a default word: "Right." Whenever she was asked anything, she just replied, "Right." This disguise could be interpreted as agreement.

Because our emotions and reactions make a lasting impact on our loved ones, even after they've forgotten our visit, being aware of how we speak and behave and being positive (smile and don't forget to breathe)[5] will improve our interactions with persons with dementia. The quality of their lives, and ours, will also improve.

Self-Care

Caring for a dependent adult with dementia is a challenge to our minds, bodies, and spirits. In order to minimize exhaustion and resentment, receive this responsibility as a call for mandatory self-care as well as an invitation to evaluate and rebalance your lifestyle and priorities. Consider adjusting to your loved one's pace. Slow down. Our culture seems to be addicted to noise and speed. Slowing down and paying attention to little things can provide a respite. Notice the birds and the flowers, and listen carefully and patiently as the person's words become harder to speak. (Breathe. Smile.) Becoming the caregiver for a person with Alzheimer's is a perfect time to learn meditation, to practice centering prayer, or to begin walking or exercising daily. It might seem impossible to add self-care to an already busy life, now made busier because of the time and attention needed to care for a person with Alzheimer's. It's not impossible to add self-care, but doing so requires a willingness to change priorities. New parents change priorities all the time when a baby arrives. Later in life, we tend not to expect that we'll need to make radical changes again to care for others. Alzheimer's disease radically shakes up our existing patterns. If we keep our minds and hearts open, adjusting our priorities to meet the new, the ever-changing needs of our loved ones and ourselves can be life-giving!

One important reason that my relationship with my mother after the onset of Alzheimer's brought me such deep healing was that Mom made no demands on me. Of course, as the disease progressed, she couldn't make demands on me or on anyone. This circumstance allowed me the opportunity and the control I needed to meet my own needs while simultaneously doing my best to meet hers. Because Alzheimer's caregiving can be physically, mentally, and emotionally exhausting, even when our loved ones are in nursing homes, I learned that self-care is the most critical practice for caregivers. There were possibly times, many of them, when Mom needed me by her side or wanted me there for company, but because she couldn't communicate this to me, I wasn't tormented over the choice of meeting her needs or my own. This free practice of self-care, unimpeded by pressure from someone else to be or to do more than I could, greatly enhanced my ability to be present with Mom and increased my joy in taking care of her. Sometimes it's actually the hardest choice to take care of our own needs, particularly when another's seem greater or more important.

We need to give ourselves permission to set and maintain healthy boundaries. For example, a man at a workshop shared how frustrated and exhausted his mother was becoming because his father, who has Alzheimer's, was constantly calling her from the nursing home and demanding that she come to pick him up and take him home. This is an opportunity for the wife to take care of herself by screening her calls and talking with her husband only once a day, if that's what she can handle. It sounds radical, I know. But talking with him once from a joyful place will be more helpful to everyone than reluctantly taking eight phone calls a day, arguing about whether she will pick him up, making up stories about the car being in the shop, and feeling frustrated, angry, and resentful.

To acknowledge and ask for help is also a practice of self-care. When a loved one is in great need, it seems wrong to focus on ourselves. The stress of long-term caregiving can put caregivers' health and well-being in jeopardy, however, so giving our needs importance—not through a selfish motivation, but from a place of self-love—will benefit everyone.

Facts about Alzheimer's Disease and Dementia

The following information is excerpted from the Alzheimer's Association website and has been adapted by the author. Dementia is not a specific disease but a word to describe a set of symptoms that result from damaged brain tissue. A number of diseases fall into this category, and this class of disease is currently being referred to as Alzheimer's Disease and Related Disorders (ADRD).

Alzheimer's Disease. Sixty to eighty percent of dementias are of the Alzheimer's type. This disease is *not* a normal function of aging. It is degenerative, terminal, and of varying duration. Often referred to as "death in slow motion," Alzheimer's can persist for four to twenty years. There is a predictable process of diminishment and decline, with brain cells dying off following the exact pattern in which they originally developed. The functioning of the patient resembles the developmental growth process in reverse.

Vascular Dementia. It is the second most common expression of dementia and is the result of a stroke. We may be able to help this type of dementia from getting worse by practicing healthy heart behaviors, including dietary changes and exercise.

Mixed Dementia. Alzheimer's disease with vascular dementia. Healthy heart behaviors can help to prevent future transient ischemic attacks, also known as TIAs (small strokes, which often cause vascular dementia), but Alzheimer's is progressive.

Frontal Lobe Dementia. A rare form of dementia. One example is Pick's disease. This disease is easier to diagnose; frontal and temporal lobes shrink and show up on brain images. It also has a rapid onset.

Lewy Body Disease. This form of dementia results from abnormal deposit of proteins in the brain. It has a more volatile presentation (such as acting out dreams, vividly and violently) and resembles Parkinson's disease.

Other diseases with symptoms of dementia include Parkinson's disease, Huntington's disease, and HIV.

Parkinsonian Dementia. Not all people with Parkinson's disease will develop dementia; those most likely to develop dementia symptoms are those who get Parkinson's disease later in life. Stiff limbs is a defining symptom.

Alcohol-Induced Dementia. Often overlooked as a source of intellectual loss, alcohol-induced dementia is considered by some to be the third or fourth most common type of dementia. It resembles other types of dementia, with common symptoms that include memory problems, language impairment, and difficulty performing motor tasks. Psychiatric symptoms, such as apathy, irritability, and resistance, are common to frontal lobe damage caused by alcohol overuse.[2]

Alzheimer's has become the catch-all word to describe the diseases of dementia. It is important to note, however, that there are different diseases and disease processes involved. Doctors, particularly neurologists, can be helpful in diagnosing the various diseases of dementia. Accurate diagnosis is crucial. For example, antipsychotic drugs should never be used in persons with Lewy Body dementia. They are very sensitive to these drugs, and their use could result in early death.

In the United States, it is estimated that there are 5.2 million people currently living with Alzheimer's disease.

Major Symptoms of Dementia

- memory loss
- cognitive loss
- confusion
- loss of motor function
- inability to communicate verbally

Each person with Alzheimer's is unique, however. When you've met one person with Alzheimer's, *you've met one person with Alzheimer's.*

Major Stages of Alzheimer's Disease

Early Stage. Early stage symptoms include memory loss, confusion, minor noticeable changes. People in this early stage are still insightful and might still be working and living independently.

Middle Stage. The more noticeable changes in language and communicating (trouble understanding what's been said, formulating words, and picking up on cues) occur at the middle stage. Symptoms may include mood changes, shadowing (following caregivers very closely, all the time—even into the bathroom), suspicion, delusions, impaired judgment, problems with personal care and hygiene, and not initiating activities.

(Just because they are not initiating doesn't mean they don't want to or can't do something. Don't ask, "Do you want to go to music?" This will confuse them. Invite them to come with you: "It's time for music. Take my hand and we'll go together.") There are safety concerns, and lots of supervision is needed in the middle stage. These persons need help with hygiene and cuing for eating and activities. The middle stage can be the longest stage, lasting for many years, though the amount of time in each stage is unpredictable.

Late Stage. Verbal communication becomes difficult, so it is important to seek ways to connect and communicate physically and emotionally with these persons. Persons in late-stage dementia will be dependent for physical cares. Ambulating becomes difficult for them. Loss of bladder/bowel control is likely. Because the brain controls everything in our bodies, capacity for physical activities like drinking, moving arms, and going down steps will be compromised.

End Stage. During the last six to twelve months, the person is incredibly compromised, possibly bed-ridden, and will ultimately forget how to swallow. This forgetting will lead to death.

For more information about Alzheimer's disease and other diseases with symptoms of dementia, call the Alzheimer's Association at 1-800-272-3900 or go to http://alz.org/index.asp.

For Further Reading

Alterra, Aaron [Elliot Stanley Goldman]. *The Caregiver: A Life with Alzheimer's.* Ithaca, NY: Cornell Paperbacks, 2007.

Armstrong, Karen. *Twelve Steps to a Compassionate Life.* New York: Alfred A. Knopf, 2011.

Bender, Sue. *Everyday Sacred: A Woman's Journey Home.* New York: HarperCollins, 1995.

Benson, Herbert, with Miriam Z. Klipper. *The Relaxation Response.* New York: HarperTorch, 2000.

Callone, Patricia R., and Connie Kudlacek, eds. *The Alzheimer's Caregiving Puzzle: Putting Together the Pieces.* New York: Demos Health, 2011.

Chödrön, Pema. *When Things Fall Apart: Heart Advice for Difficult Times.* Boston: Shambala, 1997.

Coste, Joanne Koenig. *Learning to Speak Alzheimer's: A Groundbreaking Approach for Everyone Dealing with the Disease.* New York: Houghton Mifflin, 2003.

Doidge, Norman. *The Brain That Changes Itself: Stories of Personal Triumph from the Frontiers of Brain Science*. New York: Penguin Books, 2007.

Genova, Lisa. *Still Alice*. New York: Simon & Schuster, 2009.

Hoblitzell, Olivia Ames. *Ten Thousand Joys and Ten Thousand Sorrows: A Couple's Journey through Alzheimer's*. New York: Penguin Books, 2010.

Kabat-Zinn, Jon. *Full Catastrophe Living: Using the Wisdom of Your Body and Mind to Face Stress, Pain, and Illness*. New York: Delacorte Press, 1990.

Keen, Sam. *To Love and Be Loved*. New York: Bantam, 1999.

Kleinman, Arthur. "On Caregiving." *Harvard Magazine* (July–August 2010): 25–29. http://harvardmagazine.com/2010/07/on-caregiving.

Kushner, Harold. *When Bad Things Happen to Good People*. New York: Anchor Books, 2004.

Levine, Stephen. *Unattended Sorrow: Recovering from Loss and Reviving the Heart*. Kutztown, PA: Rodale, 2005.

Madson, Patricia Ryan. *Improv Wisdom*. New York: Bell Tower, 2005.

McFadden, Susan H., and McFadden, John T. *Aging Together: Dementia, Friendship, and Flourishing Communities*. Baltimore: The Johns Hopkins University Press, 2011.

McKim, Donald K., ed. *God Never Forgets: Faith, Hope, and Alzheimer's Disease.* Louisville: Westminster John Knox Press, 1997.

Nhat Hanh, Thich. *Being Peace.* Berkeley: Parallax Press, 2005.

Parenteau, Pierre. "Communication with Alzheimer Patients: A Matter of Time, Caring and Contact." *Canadian Alzheimer Disease Review* (November 2000): 5–7. www.stacommunications. com/customcomm/back-issue_pages/ad_review/adPDFs/november2000/05.pdf.

Post, Stephen G. *The Moral Challenge of Alzheimer Disease: Ethical Issues from Diagnosis to Dying.* 2nd ed. Baltimore: The Johns Hopkins University Press, 2000.

Power, G. Allen. *Dementia Beyond Drugs: Changing the Culture of Care.* Baltimore: Health Professions Press, 2010.

Raia, Paul. "Habilitation Therapy: A New Star Scape." In *Enhancing the Quality of Life in Advanced Dementia*, edited by Ladislav Volicer and Lisa Bloom-Charette, 21–36. Philadelphia: Brunner/Mazel-Taylor Francis Group, 1999. www.nhqualitycampaign.org/files/Habilitation_Therapy_a_New_Starscape2.edit.pdf.

Richards, Marty. *Caresharing: A Reciprocal Approach to Caregiving and Care Receiving in the Complexities of Aging, Illness or Disability.* Woodstock, VT: Skylight Paths, 2009.

Rohr, Richard. *Falling Upward: A Spirituality for the Two Halves of Life.* San Francisco: Jossey-Bass, 2011.

Shenk, David. *The Forgetting—Alzheimer's: Portrait of an Epidemic.* New York: Anchor Books, 2003.

Silverstein, Nina. *Improving Hospital Care for Persons with Dementia.* New York: Springer Publishing, 2006.

Steindl-Rast, Brother David. *Gratefulness, the Heart of Prayer: An Approach to Life in Fullness.* Mahwah, NJ: Paulist Press, 1984.

Taylor, Jill Bolte. *My Stroke of Insight: A Brain Scientist's Personal Journey.* New York: Plume, 2009.

Thibault, Jane Marie, and Richard L. Morgan. *No Act of Love Is Ever Wasted: The Spirituality of Caring for Persons with Dementia.* Nashville: Upper Room Books, 2009.

Notes

Introduction

1   Marcus Borg, *Meeting Jesus Again for the First Time: The Historical Jesus and the Heart of Contemporary Faith* (San Francisco: HarperCollins, 1995), 32-33, 42.

2   Rainer Maria Rilke, *Book of Hours: Love Poems to God*, trans. Anita Barrows and Joanna Macy (New York: Riverhead Books, 2005), 88.

In the Beginning

1   Richard Rohr, *Falling Upward: A Spirituality for the Two Halves of Life* (San Francisco: Jossey-Bass, 2011), 82–86. Rohr discusses what he describes as "the most problematic lines" of the New Testament, Luke 14:26 (NRSV): "Whoever comes to me and does not hate father and mother, wife and children, brothers and sisters, yes, and even life itself, cannot be my disciple." Rohr cites the lives of Buddha and Jesus as examples of leaving home and rejecting "business as usual."

2   David Shenk, *The Forgetting: Alzheimer's: Portrait of an Epidemic* (New York: Anchor Books, 2003), 258.

3   Alan Jones, *The Soul's Journey: Exploring the Three Passages of the Spiritual Life with Dante as a Guide* (San Francisco: Harper Collins, 1995), 6.

4   Joanne Koenig Coste, *Learning to Speak Alzheimer's: A Groundbreaking Approach for Everyone Dealing with the Disease* (New York: Houghton Mifflin, 2003), 32-34.

5   Paul Raia, "Habilitation Therapy: A New Starscape," in *Enhancing the Quality of Life in Advanced Dementia,* edited by Ladislav Volcer and Lisa Bloom-Charette (Philadelphia: Brunner/Mazel-Taylor & Francis Group, 1999), 32–34. Dr. Raia's complete chapter can be accessed at www .nhqualitycampaign.org/files/Habilitation_Therapy_a_ New_Starscape2.edit.pdf

6   Coste, 32–34. Joanne Koenig Coste and Paul Raia, vice president of Clinical Programs for the Alzheimer's Association, Massachusetts/New Hampshire Chapter, created a treatment plan for persons with dementia called Habilitation Therapy. Coste defines *habilitation* as "an approach to caring for a person with progressive dementia that focuses on validating the patient's underlying emotions, maintaining dignity, creating moments for success, and using all remaining skills" (204). "The literal meaning of habilitate is 'to clothe or to dress,' but [Coste uses] it in the sense of 'to make capable,' which is an older meaning of the word" (7–8).

     Raia describes the goal of habilitation therapy as "deceptively simple—to bring about a positive emotion and to maintain that emotional state throughout the day" (Raia, 23).

7   Raia, 22-23, 29. The six critical areas referred to by Raia and Coste as "domains" are the physical domain, the social domain, the functional domain, the communication domain, the perpetual domain, and the behavioral domain (Raia, 23-36).

8   Coste, 32–34. In this interaction, the aide met Mary in her improvised reality rather than attempting to correct Mary. Her feelings were noticed and validated; for example, her feeling of loneliness and her need for nurturing were evidenced by her asking for her mother. The aide also bypassed a situation in which Mary could have felt a sense of failure. In taking this approach, the aide manifested the habilitation approach: Know that communication is possible, live in the patient's world, and enrich the patient's life.

9   Coste, 6.

10   Coste, 8.

11   Keith Johnstone, *IMPRO: Improvisation and the Theatre* (New York: Routledge, 1992), 92.

12   Rohr, 142.

13   Johnstone, 88.

14   Katie Goodman, *Improvisation for the Spirit: Live a More Creative, Spontaneous, and Courageous Life Using the Tools of Improv Comedy* (Naperville, IL: SourceBooks, Inc., 2008), 131.

15   Michelle S. Bourgeois, "Unlocking the Silent Prison: Strategies for Communicating with Persons with Dementia" (lecture, Memory Loss Conference, Southern Illinois University School of Medicine, Springfield, IL, November 8, 2011). Bourgeois is a professor of speech pathology at The Ohio State University. Her book, *Memory Books and Other Graphic Cueing Systems: Practical Communication and Memory Aids for Adults with Dementia*, offers helpful guidance for maintaining speech and engagement in persons with dementia.

16   Tom Kitwood and Kathleen Bredin, "Towards a Theory of Dementia Care: Personhood and Wellbeing," in *Ageing and Society* 12 (1992): 269-87. Kitwood and Bredin describe the following indicators of well-being in people with severe dementia:
   - the assertion of will or desire, usually in the form of dissent despite various coaxings
   - the ability to express a range of emotions
   - initiation of social contact (for instance, a person with dementia has a small toy dog that he treasures and places it before another person with dementia to attract attention)
   - affectional warmth (for instance, a woman wanders back and forth in the facility without much sociality but when people say hello to her she gives them a kiss on the cheek and continues her wandering)
   - social sensitivity in the form of a smile or taking another's hand
   - self-respect (for instance, a woman who has defecated on the floor in the sitting room attempts to clean up after herself)

- acceptance of other persons with dementia (for instance, a fast wanderer takes the hand of a slow wanderer and leads him around)
- humor (as in the case of a technical problem with a video system when a person with severe dementia unexpectedly blurts out, "Try putting a shilling in the slot.")
- creativity and self-expression, often achieved through art, music, or therapy
- showing pleasure through smiles and laughs in an exercise event
- helpfulness (for instance, a man provides a cushion for a woman seated on the hard floor)
- relaxation (for instance, a woman with dementia who has the habit of lying on the floor curled up tensely relaxes when led to the sofa)

17 www.improvboston.com and www.improvasylum.com. Classes in improvisation are available in many areas of the country through comedy clubs, drama schools, and adult education centers. Programs designed for specifically teaching improvisation techniques to people caring for persons with Alzheimer's are available worldwide through Healing Moments, Inc. at www.healingmoments.org.

18 Raia, 32.

19 Adapted from *Jainworld.com,* www.jainworld.com/education/stories25.asp.

Into the Heart of Alzheimer's

1 Aaron Alterra, *The Caregiver: A Life with Alzheimer's* (Ithaca, NY: Cornell Paperbacks, 2007), 207. Goldman used a pseudonym, Aaron Alterra, when he first wrote this book, to protect the privacy of his wife and family.

2 David Shenk, *The Forgetting: Alzheimer's: Portrait of an Epidemic,* 12-14.

3 Shenk, 25.

4 Alzheimer's Association, "2013 Alzheimer's Disease: Facts and Figures," *Alzheimer's & Dementia* 9, no. 2 (2013): 15. This

article goes on to explain:

> This includes an estimated 5 million people age 65 and older, and approximately 200,000 individuals under age 65 who have younger-onset Alzheimer's.
>
> - One in nine people age 65 and older (11 percent) has Alzheimer's disease.
> - About one-third of people age 85 and older (32 percent) have Alzheimer's disease.
> - Of those with Alzheimer's disease, an estimated 4 percent are under age 65, 13 percent are 65 to 74, 44 percent are 75 to 84, and 38 percent are 85 or older.

It is significant to note that "only about half of those who would meet the diagnostic criteria for Alzheimer's disease and other dementias have received a diagnosis of dementia from a physician."

5   Alzheimer's Association, 5, 20.

6   Alzheimer's Association, 24.

7   Zaven Khachaturian, quoted in Shenk, 65. Khachaturian, known as the "father of Alzheimer's research in the United States."

8   T. S. Eliot, "Dry Salvages," No. 3 of *The Four Quartets*, https://www2.bc.edu/john-g-boylan/files/fourquartets.pdf

9   Alterra, 210.

10   Paul Raia, "Habilitation Therapy: A New Starscape," in *Enhancing the Quality of Life in Advanced Dementia,* edited by Ladislav Volcer and Lisa Bloom-Charette (Philadelphia: Brunner/Mazel-Taylor & Francis Group, 1999), 22. Defining Alzheimer's disease and other diseases with symptoms of dementia as "disabilities," Raia's emphasis involves "active treatment of the symptoms . . . through a careful focus on the utilization of those capacities that remain, particularly the person's psychological capacity."

11   Fred Reklau, "Theses on Healing (and Cure)," copyright © 1993. Reklau is the author of *Partners in Care: Medicine and Ministry Together* (Eugene, OR: Wipf and Stock Publishers, 2010).

12   Arthur Kleinman, "On Caregiving," in *Harvard Magazine* (July–August 2010): 25.

13   Arthur Kleinman, foreword to *The Caregiver: A Life with Alzheimer's*, by Aaron Alterra (Ithaca, NY: Cornell Paperbacks, 2007), xi.

14   Alterra, 209.

15   Kleinman, "On Caregiving," 29.

16   Ibid.

17   Robin Maas and Gabriel O'Donnell, eds., "The Traditions of Prayer in Teresa and John of the Cross," in *Spiritual Traditions for the Contemporary Church* (Nashville: Abingdon Press, 1990), 246. Teresa of Avila clarifies the goal of the spiritual journey. The final phase of spiritual development in this life is not characterized by mystical experiences but by "a constant awareness of the Trinity dwelling within, coupled with total availability to the neighbor without."

18   Sallie McFague, "God as Mother," in *Weaving the Visions: New Patterns in Feminist Spirituality,* edited by Judith Plaskow and Carol P. Christ (New York: Harper Collins, 1989), 143. In order to shift our focus away from the scientifically based *cure* and toward spiritually based *healing,* we need to act according to the definition of love that McFague describes in her essay. "Love," she writes, is "unifying and reuniting . . . destabilizing, inclusive nonhierarchical fulfillment for all." This starting point, however, necessitates what Elisabeth Schussler Fiorenza describes in her essay, "In Search of Women's Heritage," in Plaskow and Christ as a "revolutionary shift in scientific paradigm, a shift with far-reaching ramifications not only for the interpretation of the world, but also for its change" (36).

19   Joan Chittister, *Heart of Flesh: A Feminist Spirituality for Women and Men* (Grand Rapids, Mich.: Eerdmans, 1998), 3-4.

20   Joan Chittister, *Gospel Days: Reflections for Every Day of the Year* (Maryknoll, N.Y.: Orbis, 1999), February 20.

21   Kleinman, "On Caregiving," 25.

22   Kleinman, "On Caregiving," 29. Arthur Kleinman met Alzheimer's through his role as primary caregiver. He writes, "I know about the moral core of caregiving not nearly so much from my professional life as a psychiatrist and medical anthropologist, nor principally from the research literature and my own studies, but primarily because of my life of

practice as a primary caregiver."

23 Kleinman, "On Caregiving," 29.

24 Olivia Ames Hoblitzelle, *Ten Thousand Joys and Ten Thousand Sorrows: A Couple's Journey Through Alzheimer's* (New York: Penguin, 2010), 125.

25 Shenk, 222. Shenk describes the infant-like state that appears during the late stages of Alzheimer's disease: "can no longer walk without assistance, can no longer sit up without assistance, can no longer smile, can no longer hold up head . . . eyes lose their ability to focus . . . the return of infant reflexes."

26 Kleinman, "On Caregiving," 29. Sallie McFague describes God as "the giver of life, as the power of being in all being," and invites her readers to consider that God can be imaged through the metaphor of mother and of father (McFague, 142). McFague was not the first feminist to imagine God as mother. In the fourteenth century, Christian mystic Julian of Norwich publicly shared her "showings" from God. True to the feminist paradigm, Julian experienced God as relational: "I saw that God rejoices that he is our Father, and God rejoices that he is our Mother, and God rejoices that he is our true spouse, and that our soul is his beloved wife" [Julian of Norwich, *Showings*, translated by Edmund Colledge and James Walsh, (Mahwah, NJ: Paulist Press, 1978), 279. Julian freely and often shared her experiences of both God and Christ as "our loving Mother" (Julian, 293). "The Creator of all things," Julian wrote, "created everything for love, and by the same love it is preserved, and always will be without end" (Julian, 190). "Parental love," according to McFague, "is the most powerful and intimate experience we have of giving love whose return is not calculated (though a return is appreciated): It is the gift of *life as such* to others. Parental love wills life . . . parental love nurtures what it has brought into existence, wanting growth and fulfillment for all" (Julian, 143). In the context of Alzheimer's care, if we apply McFague's premise that "God as Mother is parent to *all* species and wishes all to flourish" (McFague, 143), feminist caregivers will not allow this vulnerable population to be ignored, abused, or abandoned.

27 Keen, Sam. *To Love and Be Loved* (New York: Bantam, 1999),

115.

28 Keen, 116.

29 Erich Fromm, *The Art of Loving* (New York: Harper Perennial, 2006), 5.

30 Keen, 112. Adapted from Roman mythology as told by Martin Heidegger in *Being and Time* (New York: Harper & Row, 1962).

31 Keen, 119.

32 Arthur Kleinman, "The Art of Medicine," *The Lancet*, 378 (November 5, 2011): 1621.

33 Courtney Blanchard, "Chief Wadding Hangs Up Badge," *Telegraph Herald* (Dubuque, IA), March 10, 2009, section A, 1.

34 David Steindl-Rast, *The Grateful Heart* (Boulder, CO: Sounds True Recordings, 1992), audiocassette.

35 Vaclav Havel, quoted in Stephen Sapp, "Hope: The Community Looks Forward," in *God Never Forgets: Faith, Hope, and Alzheimer's Disease*, edited by Donald K. McKim (Louisville: Westminster John Knox Press, 1997), 103.

36 Life/Work Directions offers programs in Jamaica Plain, Massachusetts. For more information, contact info@lifeworkdirections.org.

37 Justin Feinstein (clinical neuropsychologist, University of Iowa), interview, September 23, 2011, Iowa City, IA.

38 Angela L. Smith and Jennifer Harkness, "Spirituality and Meaning: A Qualitative Inquiry with Caregivers of Alzheimer's Disease," *Journal of Family Psychotherapy* 13, no. 1–2 (2002): 88, 90.

39 Kleinman, "On Caregiving," 29.

40 Julian of Norwich, "*Showings*," translated by Edmund Colledge and James Walsh (Mahwah, NJ: Paulist Press, 1978), 279.

41 William Blake, quoted in Keen, 106.

42 Pierre Teilhard de Chardin, *The Divine Milieu* (New York: Perennial Classics, 2001), 56.

43 Hoblitzelle, 120, 124.

44 Kurt Ullrich, "With Alzheimer's, Watch Keeps Ticking," *Telegraph Herald* (Dubuque, IA), September 16, 2010.

45 "As the number of people with Alzheimer's disease and

other dementias grows, spending for their care will increase dramatically. For people with these conditions, aggregate payments for health care, long-term care and hospice are projected to increase from $203 billion in 2013 to $1.2 trillion in 2050 (in 2013 dollars). Medicare and Medicaid cover about 70 percent of the costs of care" (Alzheimer's Association, "2013 Alzheimer's Disease: Facts and Figures," *Alzheimer's & Dementia,* vol. 9, issue 2 [2013], 43-52).

46   Stephen Sapp, "Memory: The Community Looks Backward," and "Hope: The Community Looks Forward," in *God Never Forgets: Faith, Hope, and Alzheimer's Disease*, edited by Donald K. McKim (Louisville: Westminster John Knox Press, 1997), 38–54, 88–104.

47   Stephen Sapp (professor and chairperson, Department of Religious Studies, University of Miami, Coral Gables, FL), interview, February 17, 2009.

48   Ezekiel 12:2 (NRSV).

49   Camp Silos, "Many Uses for Corn," www.campsilos.org/ mod3/students/c_history5.shtml.

50   Camp Silos.

51   Sue Bender, *Everyday Sacred: A Woman's Journey Home* (New York: HarperCollins, 1995), 21.

52   Bender, 21-22.

53   Bender, 22.

54   James Ellor, "Celebrating the Human Spirit," in *God Never Forgets: Faith, Hope, and Alzheimer's Disease*, edited by Donald K. McKim (Louisville: Westminster John Knox Press, 1997), 20.

55   John Dominic Crossan, quoted in Burton Mack, *A Myth of Innocence* (Minneapolis: Fortress Press, 1988), 142-143. Crossan is an Irish-American religious scholar and former Catholic priest known for co-founding the Jesus Seminar.

56   Bender, 113.

57   Antoine de Saint-Exupéry, *The Little Prince*, translated by Katherine Wood (New York: Harcourt, Brace & World, 1943), 70.

58   Pat Robertson, quoted on *World News Tonight*, ABC, aired September 15, 2011. The context for this remark

was Robertson's statement that spouses of persons with Alzheimer's could divorce them without sin. He also stated that he presumed the spouse with Alzheimer's was receiving appropriate custodial care. He acknowledged that this is a complicated question and best responded to by ethicists.

59 Robert Stern, appearing on *World News Tonight*, ABC, aired September 15, 2011.

60 Augustine of Hippo, quoted in *A Treasury of Traditional Wisdom,* edited by Whitall N. Perry (San Francisco: Harper & Row, 1986), 819.

61 Sol Rogers, submitted to Helpline of the Massachusetts/New Hampshire chapter of the Alzheimer's Association, April 30, 2008.

62 Jade Angelica, "Yes, Virginia, There Is a Santa Claus," *Journal of Pastoral Care & Counseling* 65, no. 2 (2011) 10:1-2, adapted.

63 Augustine of Hippo, *Confessions*, translated by Henry Chadwick (New York: Oxford University Press), www .goodreads.com/work/quotes/1427207-confessiones

64 Shenk, 13.

65 Judith Plaskow and Carol P. Christ, "Self in Relation," in *Weaving the Visions: New Patterns in Feminist Spirituality*, edited by Judith Plaskow and Carol P. Christ (New York: HarperCollins, 1989), 173.

66 Richard Rohr, *True Self/False Self* (Cincinnati: St. Anthony Messenger Press, 2003), cassettes. Rohr claims Descartes was just being "consistent," since the West defines itself by "thinking." "After a while," Rohr continues, "We think we are our thinking, and this is the hardest thing to disassociate from . . . You cannot experience your deepest level of being or consciousness or the True Self . . . through your head."

67 Antonio Damasio, *Descartes' Error: Emotion, Reason, and the Human Brain* (New York: Penguin, 2005).

68 Plaskow and Christ, 173.

69 Citing the language used by D. H. J. Davis ("Dementia: Sociological and Philosophical Constructions," *Social Science and Medicine,* No. 58, 369-78), Stephan Millet writes, "If we take a view that people with dementia are in the process of losing their 'self' then the end result of the process of loss

is a non-person an ontological nullpoint . . . Moving away from a view of dementia in which the self is disintegrating has the potential to provide some solace to family carers" ("Self and Embodiment: A Biophenomenological Approach to Dementia," *Dementia* [June 15, 2011], 1, 12). The premise of *Where Two World's Touch* echoes Davis' conclusion: Helping caregivers to "let go of the idea of the 'person' with dementia as an ontological unit in decay, and understand that their loved one is, in effect, continuing the process of creating a life-world through the changed perceptions that come with dementia" (12). *Ontology* is the study of the nature of being or existence.

70 Plaskow and Christ write, "The notion of self as relational is prominent in feminist thinking." They explain that twentieth-century feminists challenge Descartes's position "that selfhood is to be found in the rational self-reflection of the isolated ego." Feminist thinkers are "united in their insistence that the self is essentially *embodied, passionate, relational* and *communal.* . . . they affirm that knowledge arises from the body-mind continuum, which includes passions and feelings as well as thinking. They assert that the self cannot exist apart from relationship. And they insist that identity is found in community" (173). Feminist Beverly Wildung Harrison writes, "If we begin, as feminists must, with 'our bodies, ourselves,' we recognize that all our knowledge . . . is body-mediated knowledge. All knowledge is rooted in our sensuality. We know and value the world, *if* we know and value it, through our ability to touch, to hear, to see. *Perception* is foundation to *conception.* Ideas are dependent on our sensuality. Feeling is the basic bodily ingredient that mediates our connectedness to the world. All power, including intellectual power, is rooted in feeling" ("The Power of Anger in the Work of Love," in Plaskow and Christ, 218).

71 Robert Stern, quoted in Neil Munshi, "A Healing Touch," *Boston Globe,* August 10, 2008.

72 Damasio, xix.

73 Justin S. Feinstein et al., "Sustained Experience of Emotion after Loss of Memory in Patients with Amnesia," *Proceedings of the National Academy of Sciences of the United States of America*

107, no. 17 (April 27, 2010): 7674–7679.

74 Paul Raia, "Habilitation Therapy: A New Starscape," in *Enhancing the Quality of Life in Advanced Dementia*, edited by Ladislav Volcer and Lisa Bloom-Charette (Philadelphia: Brunner/Mazel–Taylor & Francis Group, 1999), 31.

75 Damasio, xix.

76 Damasio, xi.

77 Steven Sabat and Rom Harre, "The Construction and Deconstruction of Self in Alzheimer's Disease," *Aging and Society* 12 (1992): 443–61. Sabat and Harre argue that "so-called loss of self is contingent on the failure of those around a person with dementia to respond positively to fragile clues of selfhood. As an organizing center, the self 'is not lost even in much of the end stage of the disease'"

78 Michelle S. Bourgeois, "Unlocking the Silent Prison: Strategies for Communicating with Persons with Dementia" (lecture, Memory Loss Conference, Southern Illinois University School of Medicine, Springfield, IL, November 8, 2011). Bourgeois is professor of Speech Pathology at Ohio State University. Her book, *Memory Books and Other Graphic Cueing Systems: Practical Communication and Memory Aids for Adults with Dementia*, offers helpful guidance for maintaining speech and communicative engagement in persons with dementia.

79 Dale Carnegie, *How to Win Friends and Influence People*— Principle #6. http://blog.dalecarnegie.com/uncategorized/dale-carnegies-secrets-of-success-remember-that-a-persons-name-is-to-that-person-the-sweetest-and-most-important-sound-in-any-language/.

80 "AD [Alzheimer's Disease] patients are whole individuals and can still surprise us with their ability to communicate.... Most people suffering from AD retain their capacity to understand simple language, as well as their ability to follow clear and concise instructions" (Pierre Parenteau, "Communication with Alzheimer's Patients: A Matter of Time, Caring and Contact," *Canadian Alzheimer Disease Review* [November 2000]: 7).

81 G. Allen Power, *Dementia beyond Drugs: Changing the Culture of Care* (Baltimore: Health Professions Press, 2010), 3.

82 Teresa of Avila, *Interior Castle*, translated and edited by E. Allison Peers (Mineola, NY: Dover Publications, 2007), 150, 146.

83 Tom Kitwood refers to Martin Buber's *I and Thou*: "Even when cognitive impairment is very severe, an I-Thou form of meeting and relating is often possible" (Tom Kitwood, *Dementia Reconsidered: The Person Comes First* [London: Open University Press, 1997], 12).

84 Teresa, 49. Teresa's understanding was "occupied with God and recollected in [God]," but her thoughts, "on the other hand, [were] confused and excited" (50). Italics added.

85 Teresa, 49. Kleinman quotes Emmanuel Levinas, a twentieth-century French philosopher and Talmudic commentator, as another voice with feminist undertones of relationality challenging his countryman Descartes. According to Kleinman, Levinas "insists that the ethical must always precede the epistemological or ontological in human relationships. How we know and what our being is about take second place to the affirmation of the other and responses to the other's suffering" (Kleinman, foreword to Aaron Alterra, *The Caregiver: A Life with Alzheimer's* [Ithaca, N.Y.: Cornell Paperbacks, 2007], xi).

86 Keen, 3.

87 Stephan Millett, "Self and Embodiment: A Biophenomen-ological Approach to Dementia," *Dementia* (June 15, 2011), 12.

88 Hoblitzelle, 60. In her discussion of "the grace of diminish-ment," Hoblitzelle summarizes and paraphrases Teilhard de Chardin.

89 Desiderius Erasmus, quoted in Kelly Conkling Schneider, *Prayer of the Heart: A Journey Through the Heart with Visual Prayer* (New York: Morehouse Publishing, 2006), 24. This quotation is often credited to psychologist, Carl Jung.

90 Supporting this type of connection, Maurice Friedman writes, "Only when one really listens—when one becomes personally aware of the 'signs of address' that address one not only in the words of but in the very meeting with the other—does one attain to that sphere of the 'between' that Buber

holds to be the 'really real'" (introduction to Martin Buber, *Between Man and Man* [New York: Collier Books, 1965], xv).

91 Maulana Jalal al-Din Rumi, "The Most Alive Moment," in *The Soul of Rumi: A New Collection of Ecstatic Poems*, translated by Coleman Barks (New York: HarperCollins, 2002).

92 Millett, 12.

93 James Ellor, "Celebrating the Human Spirit," in *God Never Forgets: Faith, Hope, and Alzheimer's Disease*, edited by Donald K. McKim (Louisville: Westminster John Knox Press, 1997), 15.

94 Keith Johnstone, *IMPRO: Improvisation and the Theatre* (New York: Routledge, 1992), 100.

95 Arthur Kleinman, "On Caregiving," *Harvard Magazine*, July–August 2010, 25. For those who don't feel willing or able to actively care *for* their parent, spouse, relative, or friend (for any number of reasons), one option is to care *about* him or her by choosing a qualified, caring, professional guardian and/or conservator.

96 Ellor, 17.

97 "Brooke Astor Trial Verdict Latest in Long Family Drama," *20/20*, ABC, aired October 8, 2009; "Elder Abuse Is Not Limited Just to Rich Like Brooke Astor," op-ed, *Patriot-News*, November 4, 2009, www.PennLive.com.

98 "Brooke Astor Trial Verdict."

99 The attitude that elder abuse cases are family matters and should be resolved within the family is disheartening and reminiscent of antiquated social service attitudes from twenty-five years ago regarding child abuse allegations.

100 James Ellor, "Love, Wisdom, and Justice: Transcendent Caring," in *God Never Forgets: Faith, Hope, and Alzheimer's Disease*, edited by Donald K. McKim (Louisville, Westminster John Knox Press, 1997), 59.

101 National Center on Elder Abuse, United States Administration on Aging, www.ncea.aoa.gov.

102 Stephen Post, *The Moral Challenge of Alzheimer Disease: Ethical Issues from Diagnosis to Dying*, 2d ed. (Baltimore: The Johns Hopkins University Press, 2000), 26.

103 E. T. Lucas, "Elder Abuse and Its Recognition Among Health Service Professionals," in *The Elderly in America* (New York: Garland, 1991).

104 Post, 26.

105 Lois Moorman and Sally Petrone, "Elder Abuse and Neglect Laws: Protecting Older Adults" (lecture, Memory Loss Conference, Southern Illinois University School of Medicine, Springfield, IL, November 7, 2011).

106 Eric Metaxas, *Bonhoeffer: Pastor, Martyr, Prophet, Spy* (Nashville: Thomas Nelson, Inc., 2010), inside back cover. Dietrich Bonhoeffer was killed by the Nazis in 1945 for his resistance against Hitler.

107 As Sam Keen explored the sacred relationship between love and care, he noted that in our society, care is most often defined in burdensome ways. Based on this understanding, Keen noticed that we rely more and more on "caring professionals," whom he refers to as "care-sellers" (116). Although his observations are stunningly accurate, applying this term to the professionals who care for the vulnerable population of persons with Alzheimer's causes me to shudder.

108 See Helga Niesz, "Nursing Home 'Green Houses,'" State of Connecticut General Assembly, http://cga.ct.gov/2005/rpt/2005-R-0618.htm for information about the "Green House" approach to elder care in nursing homes. See "Nursing Homes Create Home-Like, Resident-Focused Environment and Culture, Leading to Better Quality and Financial Performance, Higher Resident Satisfaction, and Lower Staff Turnover," Agency for Healthcare Research and Quality, U.S. Department of Health and Human Services, www.innovations.ahrq.gov/content.aspx?id=2621, for information about "neighborhood" designs in long-term care centers.

109 Marcus Borg translates Luke 6:36 as: "Be compassionate as God is compassionate" (replacing *merciful*, the word in the New Revised Standard Version of the Bible, with *compassionate*). According to Borg, "Compassion is not only the fruit of transformation, but the sign/mark/test of authentic Christian transformation" ("Redeeming Christian Language" [lecture,

Wartburg Theological Seminary, Dubuque, IA, October 15, 2009]).

110 Simone de Beauvoir, quoted in David Keck, *Forgetting Whose We Are: Alzheimer's Disease and the Love of God* (Nashville: Abington, 1996), 16.

111 Carl said, "It's important that we care for these people, that we don't discard them and throw them in a ditch because they are vulnerable and in need. One important reason a society cares for its people is that it helps us all to trust that we too will be cared for."

112 Marty Richards, *Caresharing: A Reciprocal Approach to Caregiving and Care Receiving in the Complexities of Aging, Illness or Disability* (Woodstock, VT: SkyLight Paths, 2009), 44.

Spirit-Inspired Caring

1   Marcus Borg, *Meeting Jesus Again for the First Time: The Historical Jesus and the Heart of Contemporary Faith* (San Francisco: HarperCollins, 1995), 125-126. Jesus scholar Marcus Borg analyzes the Hebrew Bible story of exile and return in the context of an iconic journey story for humanity. "As a life of being separated from that to which one belongs," he writes, "exile is often marked with grief." He cites Psalm 137:1: "By the rivers of Babylon, there we sat down and wept when we remembered Zion." Borg also indicates, again from Psalm 137, that "the experience of exile can also generate intense anger" (139).

For biblical descriptions of the exile, see Isaiah 40–55 (for the good news of the return), Psalm 137, and the Book of Lamentations, "which describes the suffering, despair, and angst of the generation living after the destruction of Jerusalem and the temple" (138).

2   Borg, 127.

3   Keen, 116.

4   Shams al-Din Hafiz, "Absolutely Clear," from the Penguin publication *The Subject Tonight Is Love: Sixty Wild and Sweet Poems of Hafiz*, © 1996 and 2002 Daniel Ladinsky and used with his permission.

5 Janet Ramsey, "Spiritual Resilience and Aging" (lecture, Tri-State Forum, Wartburg Theological Seminary, Dubuque, IA, October 12, 2012).

6 James Gordon, *Manifesto for a New Medicine* (Reading, MA: Perseus, 1996), 104. Carolyn Myss takes Gordon's thought a step further. She concludes that, even during difficult times, we are so afraid of change that we link our energy with the "saboteur archetype" and go into denial. Therefore, we don't actually allow ourselves to know just how *not* well things are going (Carolyn Myss, with Michael Toms, *Healing with Spirit* [Carlsbad, CA: Hay House Audio, 1997], audiocassettes). The early Christian father Evagrius Ponticus described this archetype as temptations "experienced at the hand of the demons" (quoted in Anselm Gruen, *Heaven Begins within You: Wisdom from the Desert Fathers* [New York: Crossroad, 1999], 60). St. Ignatius referred to the saboteur archetype as "the enemy" whose tactic is "to put before [people] illusory gratifications, prompting them to imagine sensual delights and pleasures, the better to hold them and make them grow in their vices and sins" (Jules Toner, *Spirit of Light or Darkness? A Casebook for Studying Discernment of Spirits* [St. Louis: The Institute of Jesuit Sources, 1995], 5.)

7 Jalal al-Din Rumi, Quatrain 91, in *Open Secret: Versions of Rumi*, translated by John Moyne and Coleman Barks (Putney, VT: Threshold Books, 1984), 5.

8 Richard Rohr, *The Spirituality of Imperfection* (Cincinnati: St. Anthony Messenger Press, 1997), audiocassette. Rohr paraphrases Heschel.

9 Richards, 83–117.

10 Deuteronomy 30:19 (NRSV).

11 Richard J. Foster, introduction to Thomas R. Kelly, *Testament of Devotion* (New York: Harper, 1941), vii–x.

12 Foster, viii.

13 Foster, ix–x.

14 Foster, x.

15 Maurice Friedman, *Martin Buber: The Life of Dialogue,* 3rd ed. (Chicago: University of Chicago Press, 1976), 139–140.

16 Martin Buber, *I and Thou*, translated by Ronald Gregor Smith

(New York: Collier, 1987), 11.

17   Matthew 15:21–28 (NRSV).

18   David V. Powers et al., "Coping and Depression in Alzheimer's
     Caregivers: Longitudinal Evidence of Stability," *Journal of
     Gerontology: Psychological Sciences* 57B, no. 3 (2002): 206.

19   Stephen Pattison, *Shame: Theory, Therapy, Theology* (New York:
     Cambridge University Press, 2000), 53.

20   J. E. Earl Thompson, Jr., "Pastoral and Clinical Implications
     of Shame" (lecture, Andover Newton Theological School,
     Newton, MA, October 5, 2010). Dr. Thompson summarizes
     the extensive work on shame by sociologist Thomas Scheff
     and psychotherapist Suzanne Retzinger, both of whom were
     influenced by Helen Block Lewis, one of the first psychoanalysts
     to write about shame. Beverly Wildung Harrison writes, "It
     is within the power of human love to build up dignity and
     self-respect in each other or to tear each other down. We
     are better at the latter than the former. However, literally
     through acts of love directed to us, we become self-respecting
     and other-regarding persons, and we cannot be one without
     the other. If we lack self-respect, we also become the sorts
     of people who can neither see nor hear each other" ("The
     Power of Anger in the Work of Love," in *Weaving the Visions:
     New Patterns in Feminist Spirituality*, edited by Judith Plaskow
     and Carol P. Christ, [New York: HarperCollins, 1989], 218).

21   Martin Buber, *I and Thou*, translated by Ronald Gregor Smith
     (New York: Collier, 1987), 11.

22   Tom Kitwood and Kathleen Bredin, "Towards a Theory
     of Dementia Care: Personhood and Wellbeing," *Ageing and
     Society* 12 (1992): 283.

23   John Denver, "On the Wings of a Dream," from *It's About
     Time* (New York: RCA, 1983), CD.

24   Buber, 4.

25   Martin Buber, *Encounter: Autobiographical Fragments* (LaSalle,
     IL: Open Court, 1967), 3.

26   Buber, *Encounter*, 38.

27   Gerald May, *The Awakened Heart: Opening Yourself to the Love
     You Need* (New York: HarperCollins, 1993), 3.

28   Thomas Merton, *The Asian Journal*, edited by Naomi Burton

et al. (New York: New Directions, 1973), 308.

29 Martin Buber, "Replies to My Critics," in *The Philosophy of Martin Buber*, edited by P. A. Schilpp and M. Friedmann (LaSalle, IL: Open Court, 1967), 693.

30 Power, 196–97.

31 Pierre Parenteau, "Communication with Alzheimer Patients: A Matter of Time, Caring and Contact," *The Canadian Alzheimer Disease Review* (November 2000): 6.

32 Henry Miller, *Big Sur and the Oranges of Hieronymous Bosch* (New York: New Directions Publishing Corp., 1957).

33 Jane Marie Thibault and Richard Morgan, *No Act of Love Is Ever Wasted: The Spirituality of Caring for Persons with Dementia* (Nashville, TN: Upper Room Books, 2009), 29.

34 Jill Bolte Taylor, *My Stroke of Insight: A Brain Scientist's Personal Journey* (New York: Plume, 2009), 35.

35 Taylor, 41.

36 The following resources about the spiritual benefits of meditation and prayer and being present in the moment were informative and inspiring companions on my journey.
In the Buddhist tradition:
Pema Chödrön, *Awakening Compassion: Meditation Practice for Difficult Times,* (Boulder, CO: Sounds True, 1995), 6 audiocassettes with booklet.
Tara Bennett-Goleman, *Emotional Alchemy: How the Mind Can Heal the Heart*, read by the author (Rochester, NY: Audio Renaissance, 2001), 2 audiocassettes.
Thich Nhat Hanh, *The Miracle of Mindfulness: A Manual on Meditation*, translated by Mobi Ho (Boston: Beacon Press, 1987).
In the Christian tradition:
Thomas Keating, *Open Mind, Open Heart: The Contemplative Dimension of the Gospel* (New York: Continuum, 2005).
New Age teachings:
Erkhart Tolle, *The Power of Now: A Guide to Spiritual Enlightenment* (Navato, CA: New World Library, 2004).

37 The following resources about the health benefits of meditation were helpful, healing companions on my journey:
Herbert Benson, with Miriam Z. Klipper, *The Relaxation*

Response (New York: Avon, 1976).

Dean Ornish, *Love & Survival: 8 Pathways to Intimacy and Health* (New York: Harper Perennial, 1999).

Jon Kabat-Zinn, *Full Catastrophe Living: Using the Wisdom of Your Body and Mind to Face Stress, Pain, and Illness* (New York: Delta, 1991).

38 Harvard Mahoney Neuroscience Institute, "Growing the Brain through Meditation," *On the Brain* vol. 12, no. 3 (Fall 2006).

39 Mindfulness, from the Sanscrit word *smrti*, is defined by Buddhist teacher Thich Nhat Hanh as "the energy to be here and to witness deeply everything that happens in the present moment, aware of what is going on within and without" [*Living Buddha, Living Christ* (New York: Riverhead Books, 1995), 204].

40 Pema Chödrön, *Start Where You Are: A Guide to Compassionate Living* (Boston: Shambala, 1994), 4.

41 Pema Chödrön, *When Things Fall Apart: Heart Advice for Difficult Times* (Boston: Shambala, 1997), 16.

42 David Steindl-Rast, *The Grateful Heart* (Boulder: Sounds True Recordings, 1992), cassette.

43 Thibault and Morgan, 15.

44 Harold Kushner, *When Bad Things Happen to Good People* (New York: Anchor Books, 2004), 45–46.

45 Borg, *Meeting Jesus Again For the First Time*, 89.

46 Kushner, 45–46.

47 Stephen Mitchell, *The Book of Job* (New York: Harper Perennial, 1992), xvi.

48 Mitchell, xix, xxvii.

49 Borg, 88–89. According to Borg, "That change—from having heard about God with the hearing of the ear [through the scripture], to 'beholding' God, from secondhand belief to firsthand relationship—is what the alternative wisdom of Jesus is most about."

50 Kushner, 50–51.

51 Mitchell, xxi.

52 Steindl-Rast, *The Grateful Heart* (Boulder, CO: Sounds True Recordings, 1992), audiocassette.

53 David Steindl-Rast, *Gratefulness, the Heart of Prayer: An Approach to Life in Fullness* (Mahwah, NJ: Paulist Press, 1984), 182.

54 Steindl-Rast, 175–76.

55 Thich Nhat Hanh, "Walking Meditation," in *Engaged Buddhist Reader*, edited by Arnold Kotler (Berkeley: Parallax Press, 1996), 46.

56 At the Map Through the Maze dementia conference held in Massachusetts in May 2012, author and presenter Joanne Koenig Coste shared the importance of waiting for persons with dementia to find their words. In an early-stage support group Coste leads for persons with dementia, one of the male participants was asked how he was. He replied with a labored stutter, "I'm f-f-f-f-f . . . " "You're fine," another man jumped in. But the first man's face turned red, and he continued to try to speak, "No, f-f-f-f-f . . . " With patience facilitated by Coste, the man finally spoke his truth, which wasn't "fine" but "frustrated." This was an exceedingly important difference! Some "experts" will encourage caregivers to complete sentences and fill in the blank with words we think persons with dementia mean in order to relieve the stress of word finding and to take attention away from their failing abilities. But in this situation, I agree with Coste: Being patient and waiting for persons with dementia to bring forward their own words will lead to more satisfying communication and connection.

57 Steindl-Rast, 176.

58 T. S. Eliot, "Dry Salvages," No. 3 of *The Four Quartets,* https://www2.bc.edu/john-g-boylan/files/fourquartets.pdf.

59 Rohr et al., *Loving the Two Halves of Life* (lectures by Richard Rohr, Ronald Rohlheiser, and Edwina Gateley) (Albuquerque, NM: Center for Action and Contemplation, 2011), compact discs.

60 "Viktor E. Frankl," *Man's Search for Meaning* (New York: Simon and Schuster, 1984), 117.

61 Steindl-Rast, 34.

62 "Mother Marianne Cope and the Sisters of St. Francis," National Park Service, www.nps.gov/kala/historyculture/marianne.htm.

63   Robert Louis Stevenson, untitled, www.robert-louis-stevenson.org/poetry/37-songs-of-travel-1895.

64   Steindl-Rast, 27.

65   C. Robert Mesle, *Process Theology: A Basic Introduction* (St. Louis: Chalice Press, 1993), 75–79.

66   Mesle outlines three aspects of a process theology of liberation:

- God has a relational character and experiences the joy and suffering of humanity. God suffers with those who experience [pain and loss], and seeks to actualize all positive and beautiful potentials.
- God seeks the actualization of the greater good.
- God exercises relational power and not unilateral control. God cannot instantly end evil [or suffering]. God works in relational ways to help guide persons to freedom [and healing].

67   Mesle, 79.

Believing in Relationship

1   Paul Raia, "Habilitation Therapy: A New Starscape," in *Enhancing the Quality of Life in Advanced Dementia,* edited by Ladislav Volcer and Lisa Bloom-Charette (Philadelphia: Brunner/Mazel–Taylor & Francis Group, 1999).

2   N. R. Kleinfield, "Alzheimer's in the News: A Behind the Scenes Special Report: More Than Death, Fearing a Muddled Mind," *New York Times,* November 11, 2002.

3   Louise M. Eder, "Heart Memories," Kansas City Alzheimer's Disease and Related Disorders Association newsletter, Spring 1984.

4   Raia, 23.

5   Raia, 31.

6   Colleen Carroll Campbell, "Alzheimer's Kills Memories, Not Emotions," *St. Louis Post-Dispatch,* April 22, 2010, www.colleen-campbell.com/P-D_Columns/PD100422Alzheimer.htm.

7   Raia, 31.

8   Lisa Genova, "Just Say Yes-And," http://blogs.alz.org/

just-say-yes-and. Lisa Genova is the author of *Still Alice* (New York: Pocket Books, 2009), a novel about early-onset Alzheimer's disease.

9   Raia, 33.

10   Campbell.

11   Daniel Tranel, University of Iowa College of Medicine, Division of Cognitive Neuroscience, Department of Neurology, interview, Iowa City, IA, October 25, 2011. Tranel changed the actual names and locations of the persons involved to protect their privacy.

12   Justin S. Feinstein et al., "Sustained Experience of Emotion after Loss of Memory in Patients with Amnesia," *PNAS/ Proceedings of the National Academy of Sciences of the United States of America* 107, no. 17 (April 27, 2010): 7674.

13   Feinstein, 7678.

14   Ibid.

15   Feinstein, 7674.

16   Norman Doidge explains, "The hippocampus turns our short-term explicit memories into long-term explicit memories for people, places, and things—the memories to which we have conscious access.... Explicit memory consciously recollects specific facts, events, and episodes. It is the memory we use when we describe and make explicit what we did on the weekend, and with whom, and for how long. It helps us to organize our memories by time and place" (*The Brain That Changes Itself: Stories of Personal Triumph from the Frontier of Brain Science* [New York: Penguin Books, 2007], 229). Doidge compares the explicit memory system, which is supported by language, and the "procedural or implicit" memory system. Procedural/implicit memory is well-developed by the time a child is twenty-six months old and will remain functional for persons with Alzheimer's long after cognition and verbal language skills decline. He writes, "Procedural/implicit memory functions when we learn a procedure or group of automatic actions occurring outside our focused attention, in which words are not generally required. Our nonverbal interactions with people and many of our emotional memories are part of our procedural memory system" (228).

Doidge cites the work of E. R. Kandel, who says, "During the first 2–3 years of life, when an infant's interaction with its mother is particularly important, the infant relies primarily on its procedural memory systems" (E. R. Kandel, "Biology and the Future of Psychoanalysis: A New Intellectual Framework for Psychiatry Revisited," *American Journal of* Psychiatry, Vol. 156, No. 4 [1999], 505-24). Similarly, people in the later stages of Alzheimer's disease will be relying on and using their remaining capacities for experiencing procedural/implicit memories.

17 Raia, 22.
18 Joseph Campbell, interview by Bill Moyers, *The Power of Myth*, PBS, 1988.
19 Pam Belluck, "The Vanishing Mind: Giving Alzheimer's Patients Their Way, Even Chocolate," *The New York Times*, January 1, 2011, Health Section, A1.
20 A currently popular anti-psychotic drug, Abilify, is advertised on television as a compliment to anti-depressant medication. The advertisement contains a warning that Abilify may cause death for elderly patients with dementia.
21 Feinstein, 76-78.
22 Rabindrinath Tagore, "Fireflies," *Poetry Chaikhana: Sacred Poetry from Around the World*, www.poetry-chaikhana.com/T/TagoreRabind/Fireflies.htm.
23 Dietrich Bonhoeffer, *Letters and Papers from Prison* (New York: Touchstone, 1997), 3.
24 Abraham Joshua Heschel, *The Sabbath* (New York: Farrar, Straus and Giroux, 1975), 3, 6, 29.
25 Sherri Edwards, "My Mother's Unlikely Gift of Dementia," *Huffington Post*, December 8, 2011, www.huffingtonpost.com/sherri-edwards/mother-with-dementia_b_1121726.html.
26 Stephen Post, *The Moral Challenge of Alzheimer's Disease: Ethical Issues from Diagnosis to Dying*, 2d ed. (Baltimore: The Johns Hopkins University Press, 2000), 1.
27 Coleen attended college part-time for six years; during these same years, she worked full-time, parented her two sons, and cared for her mom on a regular basis. Coleen completed her

BA in business one year before her mom died.

28   David Steindl-Rast, *The Grateful Heart* (Boulder: Sounds True Recordings, 1992), audiocassette.

29   David Shenk supports Mary Anne's awareness that the losses associated with Alzheimer's disease could be worse for the caregiver than the afflicted persons: "Still, caregivers must try to understand both the frustrations and the unexpected benefits of having an unraveling mind. What they may at first presume to be a uniformly awful experience for the victims can sometimes perhaps be peculiarly satisfying and even enriching—a final intellectual and esthetic adventure. . . . Alzheimer's keeps things new. The Alzheimer's mind is constantly flooded with new stimuli; everything is always in the moment, a rich, resonant, overwhelming feeling. . . . Ever-freshness, then, may be considered an Alzheimer's consolation prize. This may be a particularly difficult idea for caregivers to swallow . . . they must suffer through the oppressive repetition. . . . in the often deadening, disheartening world of Alzheimer's care, caregivers wake up thousands of days in a row facing the same tourist wanting to take exactly the same tour" (*The Forgetting—Alzheimer's: Portrait of an Epidemic* [New York: Anchor Books, 2003]. 194-195).

30   Ione was a neighbor of Mom's at the nursing home. One night the phone at the nurses' station was ringing off the hook, and no one was answering. Finally, Ione shouted out what everyone was probably thinking: "Answer the damn phone!" When no one came to answer the phone, Ione rolled her wheelchair behind the desk and answered it herself. "Hello," she said, annoyed. "Mom?" asked a surprised Mary Anne, the caller on the other end of the phone. "Yes. Oh hello, honey!" replied a now-delighted Ione.

31   As Raia puts it, "There is an unfortunate but persistent myth that people with Alzheimer's disease, because they may not remember friends or be able to contribute to a relationship, no longer have a need for social experience and interaction. In fact, they have an increasing need for all the social benefits that derive from relationships. Victims of Alzheimer's disease may lose the ability to initiate social interaction, but not their

need for it" (26).

32   Myra Scovel, "The Wind of the Spirit," in *The Weight of A Leaf* (Philadelphia: The Westminster Press, 1970), 45.

33   Carl is paraphrasing 2 Corinthians 7:2 (NRSV).

34   Rainer Maria Rilke, *Letters to a Young Poet*, translated by M. D. Herter Norton (New York: W. W. Norton, 1962), 35.

35   Rilke, 35.

36   Michelle S. Bourgeois, "Beyond Memory Books: Effective Strategies for Communicating with Persons with Dementia" (lecture, Memory Loss Conference, Southern Illinois University Medical School, Springfield, IL, November 8, 2011).

37   Stephan Millett, "Self and Embodiment: A Biophenomenological Approach to Dementia," *Dementia* (June 15, 2011), 12. Millet writes, "People with dementia are . . . 'driven by meaning'—but without committing to cognition-reliant definitions of selfhood and intentionality."

38   Joanne Koenig Coste, *Learning to Speak Alzheimer's: A Groundbreaking Approach for Everyone Dealing with the Disease* (New York: Houghton Mifflin, 2003), 7.

39   Stephen Levine, *Unattended Sorrow: Recovering from Loss and Reviving the Heart* (Emmaus, PA: Rodale Books, 2005), 192.

40   Stephen Levine and Ondrea Levine, *Who Dies? An Investigation of Conscious Living and Conscious Dying* (New York: Anchor Books, 1989), 163.

41   Levine and Levine, 163.

42   Levine, 204.

43   G. Allen Power, *Dementia Beyond Drugs: Changing the Culture of Care* (Baltimore: Health Professions Press, 2010), 196–197; Parenteau, 6; Levine, 74.

44   "My child, be attentive to my words; incline your ear to my sayings. Do not let them escape from your sight; keep them within your heart" (Proverbs 4:20-21, NRSV).

45   Levine and Levine, 163.

46   Doidge describes the right hemisphere nonverbal capacities of the developing brain between the ages of ten months and twenty-six months, similar to those of a person in the later stages of Alzheimer's: "During the first two years of life, the

mother principally communicates nonverbally with her right
hemisphere to reach her infant's right hemisphere....The right
hemisphere generally processes nonverbal communication; it
allows us to recognize faces and read facial expressions, and it
connects us to other people. It, thus, processes the nonverbal
visual cues exchanged between a mother and her baby. It
also processes the musical component of speech, or tone, by
which we convey emotion" (226).

47 Levine, 76.

48 Levine, 74.

49 Levine and Levine, 164.

50 Levine, 196.

51 Jalal al-Din Rumi, "The Guest House," in *The Essential
Rumi*, translated by Coleman Barks with John Moyne (San
Francisco: Harper Collins, 1995), 109.

52 Jill Bolte Taylor, who suffered and recovered from a stroke,
writes, "I shifted from the doing-consciousness of my left
brain to the being-consciousness of my right brain. . . .
I stopped thinking in language and shifted to taking new
pictures of what was going on in the present moment. . . .
All I could perceive was right here, right now, and it was
beautiful. . . . The now offline intellectual mind of my left
hemisphere no longer inhibited my innate awareness that I
was the miraculous power of life . . . in the absence of my
left hemisphere's negative judgment, I perceived myself as
perfect, whole, and beautiful just the way I was. . . . Although
I could not understand the words they spoke, I could read
volumes from their facial expression, and body language. I
paid very close attention to how energy dynamics affected
me. I realized that some people brought me energy while
others took it away" [*My Stroke of Insight: A Brain Scientist's
Personal Journey* (New York: Plume, 2009) 71–77].

53 Raia cites Abraham Maslow's *Toward a Psychology of Being*
(New York: John Wiley & Sons, 1968) as a basis of habilitation
therapy. In addition, Raia applies Maslow's humanistic
perspective to persons with Alzheimer's and dementia (22).

54 Mark 14:33–34 (NRSV).

55 Jane Thibault and Richard Morgan, *No Act of Love Is Ever*

Wasted: The Spirituality of Caring for Persons with Dementia (Nashville, TN: Upper Room Books, 2009), 111.

56 Sister Catherine Griffiths, my spiritual director. This is her interpretation of Christian mystic Julian of Norwich's thoughts about death (June 2007).

Looking Back, Walking On

1 David Steindl-Rast, The Grateful Heart (Boulder, Sounds True Recordings, 1992), audiocassette.

2 Richard Rohr et al., *Loving the Two Halves of Life* (lectures by Richard Rohr, Ronald Rohlheiser, and Edwina Gateley (Albuquerque, NM: Center for Action and Contemplation, 2011), audio compact discs.

3 Dennis Linn, Sheila Fabricant Linn, and Matthew Linn, *Don't Forgive Too Soon: Extending the Two Hands That Heal* (Mahwah, NJ: Paulist Press, 1997); Marie M. Fortune, "Forgiveness: The Last Step," in *Violence Against Women and Children: A Christian Theological Sourcebook*, ed. Carol J. Adams and Marie M. Fortune (New York: Continuum, 1995), 201-6.

4 Fortune, 204; Ellen Bass and Laura Davis, *The Courage to Heal: A Guide for Women Survivors of Child Sexual Abuse,* 3d ed. (New York: HarperCollins, 1994), 162.

5 Robert L. Browning and Roy A. Reed cite the *process model of forgiveness* developed by Robert D. Enright, indicating that there are several challenging steps:
    1. Experience negative psychological consequences of the injury
    2. Recognize a need for resolution
    3. Deciding between justice and mercy as a strategy
    4. Identify your forgiveness motive
    5. Make a decision to forgive
    6. Execute internal forgiveness strategies
    7. Execute behavioral reconciliation strategies, culminating in release

    (*Forgiveness, Reconciliation and Moral Courage: Motives and Designs for Ministry in a Troubled World* [Grand Rapids, MI: Eerdmans, 2004], 65-9).

Professor J. Earl Thompson, Jr., quotes Enright as he writes about step 5 in the above model of forgiveness. The decision to forgive is "a moral choice based in a long and arduous process of struggle and suffering. Forgiveness is not cheap. It costs the injured dearly in emotional and spiritual pain" ("Steps Toward Forgiveness [A Process of Forgiveness]: Insights from Robert D. Enright and Terry Hargrave, modified by Professor Thompson" [lecture, Andover Newton Theological School, Newton, MA, November 9, 2010]).

6 Solomon Schimmel, *Wounds Not Healed by Time: The Power of Repentance and Forgiveness* (New York: Oxford University Press, 2002), 122, 85. Citing Mishna, Bava Kamma 8:7, Shimmel states, "The Mishnah and other rabbinic sources emphasize that the victim must forgive the offender who has appropriately repented."

7 Everett L. Worthington, Jr., *Forgiving and Reconciling: Bridges to Wholeness and Hope* (Downers Grove, IL: InterVarsity Press, 2003), 31-41.

8 Schimmel, 137.

9 Naomi Feil, *Validation: The Feil Method: How to Help Disoriented Old-Old* (Cleveland: Edward Feil Productions, 1982), 17.

10 Browning and Reed, 49.

11 J. Earl Thompson, Jr., "Forgiveness—Everett L. Worthington, Jr. and Terry Hargrave" (lecture, Andover Newton Theological School, Newton, MA, November 16, 2010). Using the forgiveness work of Hargrave as a springboard, Professor Thompson begins the discussion of reconciliation, which is essentially "a rebirth of the relationship" brought forth by the restoration of trust in relationships that have been fractured—*if* the restoration is safe and possible."

12 Janet Ramsey, "Forgiveness and Healing" (lecture, Tri-State Forum, Wartburg Theological Seminary, Dubuque, IA, April 15, 2010). Dr. Ramsey is Professor Emeritus at Luther Seminary and a Marriage and Family Counselor in St. Paul, MN.

13 J. Earl Thompson, Jr., "Steps Toward Forgiveness (A Process of Forgiveness): Insights from Robert D. Enright and Terry Hargrave, modified by Professor Thompson"

(lecture, Andover Newton Theological School, Newton, MA, November 9, 2010). This Biblical reference to a "Refiner's Fire" is from Malachi 2:17–3:60. It is possible for an injured person to discover fresh meaning for one's self and perhaps even a new purpose in life as a result of suffering and engaging in the process of forgiveness. This insight "speaks to the idea that life is loss and paradoxically gain. Being injured and experiencing numerous losses can lead us into deeper maturity and greater clarity of purpose and direction if we can turn loose of our bitterness and resentment."

14 Bass and Davis, 162.

15 Ramsey, lecture. Dr. Ramsey defined what forgiveness *is not*:
- Forgiveness is not forgetting. Remembering the harm helps you stay safe.
- Forgiveness is not minimizing.
- Forgiveness is not justifying or condoning.
- Forgiveness is not an event. It's a process.
- Forgiveness is not an act of willpower. It is not something we can command.
- Forgiveness is not universal. It's not even a goal for some.
- Forgiveness is not reconciliation. We have to stay far, far away from some people.

16 Schimmel, 123.

17 Bass and Davis, 162.

18 Ramsey, lecture. Dr. Judith Lewis Herman supports Ramsey's position that forgiveness is not a human achievement. Herman indicates that revenge fantasies and forgiveness fantasies are an "attempt at empowerment" for victims of abuse. "The survivor imagines that she can transcend her rage [through forgiveness] and erase the impact of the trauma through a wild, defiant act of love. But it is not possible to exorcise the trauma through either hatred or love. Like revenge, the fantasy of forgiveness often becomes a cruel torture because it is out of reach for most ordinary human beings" (*Trauma and Recovery: The Aftermath of Violence—From Domestic Abuse to Political Terror* [New York: Basic Books, 1992], 89–90).

19 Bass and Davis write, "Feeling compassion for another human being feels good. It often arises out of the fact that you are

feeling compassionate toward yourself, or because you have begun to view a particular family member in a different way" (162). Enright's model of forgiveness also acknowledges the importance of empathy, suggesting that the injured person must take the offender seriously and seek to understand who she is, and how she perceives and senses the world. Professor Thompson acknowledges, along with Bass, Worthington, and Enright, that "empathy is incredibly difficult for us under any circumstances" (J. Earl Thompson, Jr. [lecture, November 9, 2010]).

20 Worthington, 95-112. Worthington proposes a five-step process of forgiveness, which he names R-E-A-C-H:
Recall the hurt.
Empathize with the person who injured us.
Conceptualize forgiveness as an **A**ltruistic gift.
Commit to forgive.
Hold onto forgiveness.

21 Browning and Reed, 55.

22 J. Earl Thompson, Jr., November 30, 2010.

23 Martin Buber, *I and Thou*, trans. Ronald Gregor Smith (New York: Collier, 1987), 18.

24 George Odell, "We Need One Another," in *Singing the Living Tradition* (Boston: Unitarian Universalist Association, 1993), #468.

25 Karen Armstrong, *Twelve Steps to a Compassionate Life* (New York: Knopf, 2010), 19.

26 David Shenk, *The Forgetting Alzheimer's: Portrait of an Epidemic* (New York: Anchor Books, 2003), 225–226.

27 Armstrong, 116.

28 Armstrong, 6.

29 Sam Keen, *To Love and Be Loved* (New York: Bantam, 1999), 116.

30 Jeffrey Bishop, "A Call to Cure, A Call to Care" (lecture, Joy of Caring Conference, Clarke University, Dubuque, IA, August 17, 2013).

31 Bishop.

32 Bishop.

33 According to Bishop, the depersonalizition of patients by the

conventional medical system, particularly those who can't be cured and are dying, is the basis for burnout of health care providers.

34   Armstrong, 8.

35   Pema Chödrön, *Start Where You Are: A Guide to Compassionate Living* (Boston: Shambala, 1994), x.

36   Armstrong, 9.

37   Richard Rohr, *True Self/False Self* (Cincinnati: St. Anthony Messenger Press, 2003). audiocassettes.

38   Marcus Borg, *Meeting Jesus Again For the First Time: The Historical Jesus and the Heart of Contemporary Faith* (San Francisco: HarperCollins, 1995), 47.

39   Borg, 48–49. Borg also writes, "For Jesus, this is what God is like. . . . According to Jesus, compassion is to be the central quality of a life faithful to God the compassionate one."

40   Bishop.

41   Rohr, *True Self/False Self.*

42   "You Are So Beautiful to Me," by Bruce Fisher, Billy Preston, and Dennis Wilson, recorded by Joe Cocker on *I Can Stand a Little Rain*, Sony/ATV Music Publishing LLC, Universal Music Publishing Group, Warner/Chappell Music, Inc., 1974.

43   Through her actions, Julie was manifesting the goal of habilitation therapy. She was helping Mom to begin her day in a positive emotional state.

44   Mary Vineyard, *11th Sunday in Ordinary Time* 6/17/12, reflections on scripture readings: Ezk 17:22–24, Ps 92, 2 Cor 5:6–10, Mk 4:26–34, emailed to author.

45   Armstrong, 9-11. Armstrong identifies the four elements of love from the Buddhist tradition as *maîtri* ("loving kindness"), the desire to bring happiness to all sentient beings; *karuna* ("compassion"), the resolve to liberate all creatures from their pain; *mudita* ("sympathetic joy"), which takes delight in the happiness of others; and *upkesha* ("even-mindedness"), an equanimity that enables us to love all beings equally and impartially.

46   Armstrong, 21–22.

47   Borg, *Meeting Jesus Again for the First Time*, 49. Borg is